11262063

RENAISSANCE FICTIONS OF ANATOMY

Renaissance Fictions of Anatomy

DEVON L. HODGES

The University of Massachusetts Press
AMHERST, 1985

Library of Congress Cataloging in Publication Data

Hodges, Devon L., 1950–
Renaissance fictions of anatomy.
Bibliography: p.
Includes index.
1. English literature—Early modern, 1500–1700—
History and criticism.   2. Literary anatomies.   I. Title.
PR428.A52H6   1985   820′.9′003   84–16343
ISBN 0–87023–470–6

Publication of this book was assisted by the
American Council of Learned Societies under a grant from the
Andrew W. Mellon Foundation.

TO ERIC

Contents

*Diachylum and bandages were trailing over
the mantlepiece. The surgical case stood in
the middle of the desk, probes filled a basin
in the corner—and against the wall was a picture
of a flayed man.
Pécuchet complimented the doctor on it.
"Anatomy must be a fascinating study."*

—GUSTAVE FLAUBERT

Acknowledgments

This study of anatomies could not have been completed without the kind assistance of those who read many dissected pieces of it. I am fortunate to have friends with the critical acumen of James Bunn, Richard Fly, Murray Schwartz, and William Warner. Their advice gave this project its initial focus and their encouragement helped sustain it. Angus Fletcher's wit and encyclopedic knowledge of the Renaissance stimulated my thinking and sharpened my writing when my manuscript was nearing completion. Most of all, I am indebted to Laurence Michel. He has read and reread chapters, evaluating, tinkering with clumsy prose, and always encouraging me onward. Though there is no way to acknowledge his efforts fully, I thank him for the generous and indispensable assistance he has offered me.

I am also grateful for the suggestions I have received from other readers. Kirby Farrell and Susan Snyder carefully read the manuscript and offered criticisms that allowed me to shape my argument and to make it more vivid. Pamela Campbell, a meticulous editor, helped me refine the text in crucial ways. I would also like to thank Bruce Wilcox for his interest and advice.

Thanks are also due to my friends and family who gave me encouragement, for which I am most grateful. In particular, the intelligence, wit, and energy of the women among them has been an inspiration.

None of those who helped improve the text can be held responsible for its flaws. Mangled facts, gaps in logic, or tortured style are products of my own anatomizing technique. As did Robert Burton in his preface, "I confess my fault."

Much of the material in chapters five and six first appeared elsewhere. "Anatomy as Tragedy" is reprinted from " 'Cut Adrift and Cut to the Brains': The Anatomized World of *King Lear*," *ELR,* Spring, 1981. Most of "Anatomy as Science" is reprinted from Devon Leigh Hodges, "Anatomy as Science" in *Assays: Critical Approaches to Medieval and Renaissance Texts* (Volume I), Peggy A. Knapp and Michael Stugrin, editors, published in 1981 by the University of Pittsburgh Press. Both articles are used by permission. I am also grateful to the Library of Congress for permission to photocopy eight of the "musclemen" illustrations from the *Fabrica* of Vesalius.

RENAISSANCE FICTIONS OF ANATOMY

1 · Of Anatomy

IN THE PAST few years, talk about discourse and its transformation has assumed precision and authority. The work of Michel Foucault, in a poetic language that has often exasperated its readers, dramatically insists that our modes of knowing, our discourses, are somewhat ephemeral events.[1] But it is only recently that his story of cultural change has been documented. Timothy J. Reiss, in *The Discourse of Modernism,* refines Foucault's argument and uses the language and apparatus of the scholar. With these tools, Reiss convincingly demonstrates that our own mode of "analytico-referential" discourse emerged during the Renaissance from within a discourse of resemblance, a medieval system of "patterning."[2] But though Reiss provides extensive evidence of this transformation, his abstract discussion does not often conjure up the particular powers and kinds of anguish associated with a crisis in discourse, with the displacement of truth from within a web of language to a referent located someplace outside it.[3] In this study, I hope to get at the experience of this crisis by focusing on one group of texts, "anatomies." With these texts, where the desire for analysis confronts an older love of resemblance, I want to illuminate the passions, tortures, and pleasures associated with the difficult project of cultural transformation.

Anatomies were a fad in sixteenth-century England. Men of every persuasion wrote them. There are literary anatomies, theological anatomies, scientific anatomies. The wide range of such texts dramatically illustrates the Renaissance writer's concern to strip away false appearances and expose the truth. With violent determination, writers of anatomies used their pens as scalpels to cut through appearances and reveal the mute truth of objects.[4] This new method of articulation promised to destroy idols and false forms, and to replace them with a knowledge built on solid facts—but this promise was not fulfilled. In each of the works I explore, a writer takes on the task of looking within a form to locate its deepest truths. He seems to stand apart, objective, neutral, as he examines the body set before him. Yet, in spite of his pose of scientific detachment, the procedure of delving into forms collapses distinctions as depths are turned into ever more surfaces. The conflict within an anatomy between its desires and methods marks the anatomy as a transitional form and provides the subject of this study.

The word "anatomy" became a part of the language when the feudal body of England was decaying and a new horizon of knowledge was opening up. The word made its first significant appearance during the Tudor period: the *Oxford English Dictionary* records that it was first used to signify a dissected body in 1540; the process of dissection, 1541; the science of bodily structure, 1391 (the anomaly in this list of dates) and next in 1541; it is recorded as a trope in 1569. The shift from an analogical to an empirical order which enabled the appearance of the anatomy can be connected with social and economic events of this period—the decay of feudalism, the emergence of the bourgeoisie, the fragmentation of a unified church all accompanied the rise of scientific rationalism which put traditional beliefs in doubt. But though social and economic factors help explain the proliferation of anatomies at this time, they do not adequately account for the complexity that comes to the surface when answering the question, What is an anatomy?

At first glance the anatomist seems to desire nothing more than to portray a unified order; the work of Andreas Vesalius, the founder of modern medical anatomy, offers one demonstration of the way in which the technique provides a pathway to truth. Vesalius published *De Corporis Fabrica* in 1543, the same year that Copernicus published *On the Motion of Heavenly Bodies*—a conjunction of publishing events that has led one historian of medicine to comment that Copernicus displaced the center of the cosmos as Vesalius displaced the center of man: "Between the two they destroyed forever . . . the theory of microcosm and macrocosm."[5] Yet Vesalius insists that he is recovering the central truth of man, not displacing it. In his preface to the *Fabrica,* he emphasizes the role of anatomy as a method of teaching that will allow students to see the body unencumbered by representation, by words and books, instead of the way it is "wrongly taught in the schools." He memorably depicts the false teachers of anatomy as "jackdaws aloft their high chair, with egregious arrogance croaking things from books of others, or reading what has already been described." His text, along with illustrations that place the parts of the body "more exactly before the eyes than even the most precise language," is meant to provide students with an example of the proper way to "undertake dissection."[6] The central ambition of the anatomist is outlined here—to negate false representations of reality and present the unadorned truth to the eyes of his readers. The proper way to accomplish this, a systematic anatomy of the body, is proffered as a nondisruptive method for transmitting information lost to men through the bunglings of "arrogant jackdaws."

According to Walter Ong, efficient methods of medical instruction, like those advocated by Vesalius, played an important role in bringing about the shift from a mode of knowledge based on discoursing about first principles to a quantitative mode featuring lists, diagrams, and tables that literally "contain" knowledge. He specifically relates the vogue for anatomies to methods of medical study:

Medicine at this time [the sixteenth century] makes its own special contribution to the collection of spatial models for thought by encouraging the fad of thinking of scientific or quasi-scientific treatises as presentations of "bodies" of knowledge. It also encouraged the related fad of performing intellectual "anatomies," which are analyses or "dissections" of such "bodies" of knowledge undertaken sometimes in a friendly and sometimes in a polemic spirit.[7]

In his description of the impact medical methods of instruction had on the structure of thought and language, Ong usefully illuminates the anatomist's compulsion to produce catalogs and tables.[8] He bypasses, however, the anatomist's effort to use anatomy to arrive at the knowledge of universals. Such an omission is a necessity of the opposition Ong creates between the transcendental language of the Word and the discourse of science—an opposition that obscures the interplay of science and metaphysics within an anatomy. Anatomical truth was not based simply on the observation and enumeration of parts of a dissected body; an anatomist also claimed the ability to see how each part of the body revealed the divine purpose of its creation.

The anatomist's pursuit of the final cause of structure, and his frequent ability to find it, made him seem both a metaphysician of godlike powers and a skilled investigator of sensible phenomena. Galen, the most influential of ancient anatomists, notes in his *De Usu Partium:* "In every case the body is adapted to the character and the faculty of the soul."[9] Vesalius, following in this tradition, describes the body as the "finished product of creation most perfected" and undertakes his anatomy because it is "wretched" that "the harmony of the human body which we shall publish to the world should lie constantly concealed; that man be completely unknown to himself; and that the structure of instruments so divinely created by the Great Artificer of all things should remain unexamined. . . ."[10] Vesalius was apparently unaware that his method of making man known to himself would displace the center of man and challenge the relationship between form and meaning articulated in the theory of resemblances. How does this happen?

The illustrations in the *Fabrica* reveal the tension between the belief in the body as an ideal form and the procedures of the anatomist which describe it as an empirical object. Looking at the spectacular illustrations of Vesalius's text, one can observe the breaking up of the idealized body of man: microcosm becomes matter to be enumerated in the scientific text.[11] The science of medicine has acquired information important to its development, but we understand the soul no better when the anatomy is completed. For example, the first of the "muscle-men" illustrations depicts a man heroic in stature and demeanor.

He is huge—this is man as the measure of all things, a form containing the vastness of the universe. He stands in front of a landscape that, because of his size, he dominates almost grotesquely. Included in the background is a rural village, too small and closed-off to provide a context for the figure. In other plates the landscape is covered with ruins or is so desolate that there is even less shelter for the naked figure. The isolation and size of the body makes us conscious of its physicality, but we are still not prepared when it becomes conflated with a cadaver and the decaying natural landscape serves as an anatomical theater. In the first three plates, though muscles are revealed and letters fixed to them, we observe these superficial characteristics passively—it is not yet clear that a violent manipulation must take place to enable us to look at the depths of the body. Only in the next plates, which show tissue hanging from the figure, is it clear that surfaces are being ruined so that our eyes, like scalpels, can pierce ever further into the flesh of a man. The sixth plate is a monster, a human form distorted by the process of anatomy, and the seventh "muscleman" hangs by his neck to undergo our punishing scrutiny. Finally we reach the central truth of the body, a skeleton. It is hard to privilege this collection of bones over the surfaces that once hid it from sight—in the process of anatomy, the depths have lost their significance.

The illustrations of the *Fabrica* record and enact a violent event: the imposition of the body as object on an idealized body, the "finished body of creation most perfected." The anatomist cuts, dissects, flays, tears, and rips the body apart in order to know it.[12] The artist, however, gives this violent process a strange dignity, which is partially an acknowledgment of the anatomist's claim that fragmentation is a means of getting at a unified truth: an idealized body is destroyed, but a new field of knowledge is opened up for the creation of a scientific order of knowledge. It is also a sign that the heroic human subject of the anatomy has not been completely conquered. By the end of the "musclemen" series a skeleton is all that remains—yet the bones are poised to retain signs of human suffering. They function as *memento mori* rather than medical illustrations. In the illustrations of Vesalius's text, the idealized man of the Renaissance is not completely replaced by the dehumanized parts distributed in an anatomy textbook. As a result, the boundary between living and dead matter is significantly obscured.

Has an anatomy or a vivisection been performed? This question is provoked by the way the anatomist seems to threaten life—his painful procedure for revealing truths seems to kill them. Though he tells us that he will expose a tangible truth, the anatomist instead turns up the depths, displaces parts from a coherent whole, and flattens out bodies once full with divine significance. That significance decays as the anatomy proceeds, turning finally into fragments that are not immediately placed in a new order. No doubt the disruptive relation between anatomical parts and systematic order explains why the anatomist is suspicious of order and therefore desires to dissect it. The imbalance between parts and the whole may also explain why the anatomist is always trying to create a new more comprehensive order than any that has existed before. Thus the anatomy has a paradoxical doubleness: it is a method for revealing order, but it also causes its decay.

This doubleness is apparent in "spiritual" anatomies as well as in "scientific" ones. Early "spiritual" anatomies are ostensibly moral works designed simply to cut away sins that hide the truth from sight: their titles give evidence of their attachment to a program of purification. Augustino Mainardo, author of the first one such written in English, calls his work *An Anatomi: that is to say A parting in peeces of the Mass. Which discovereth the horrible errors, and the infinite abuses unknowen to the people, aswel of the Mass as of the Mass book* (1557).[13] Written in the interest of ecclesiastical reform, this work employs the anatomy as an aggressive critical method for studying vice and attacking it. By cutting apart vice, the anatomist cleanses a diseased body and discovers the cause of its sickness for our edification—a method of therapy explained by Ovid who writes in his *Metamorphosis:* "The wound that will not respond to medicine must be cut away."[14] But there is a danger signaled in Mainardo's title. If "abuses" are "infinite" then how can he stop short of murdering the body he dissects? His excess subverts the "objectivity" of anatomy and emphasizes its aggressive spirit. Violence is required to fragment a body, whether the purpose is to discover its secrets or to annihilate it as an obstacle to truth. One way to

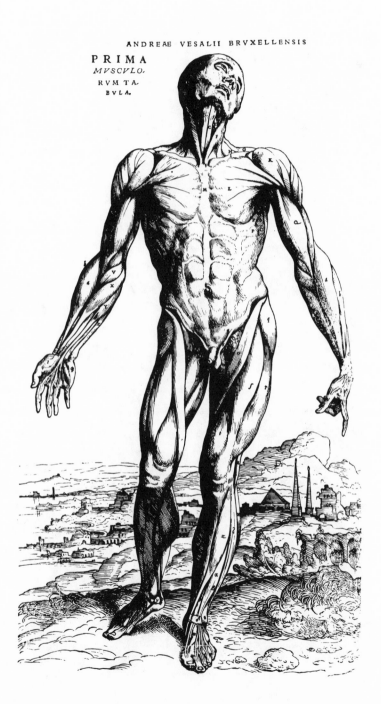

ANDREAE VESALII BRVXELLENSIS

PRIMA
MVSCVLO.
RVM TA.
BVLA.

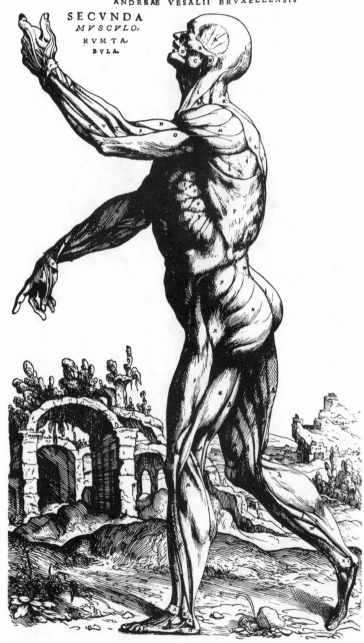

ANDREAE VESALII BRVXELLENSIS

SECVNDA
MVSCVLO.
RVM TA
BVLA.

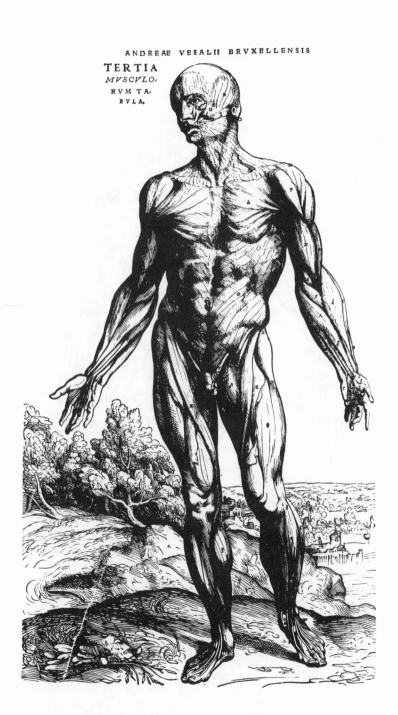

ANDREAE VESALII BRVXELLENSIS
TERTIA
MVSCVLO,
RVM TA,
BVLA.

PRIMA MVSCV-
LORVM TABVLA.

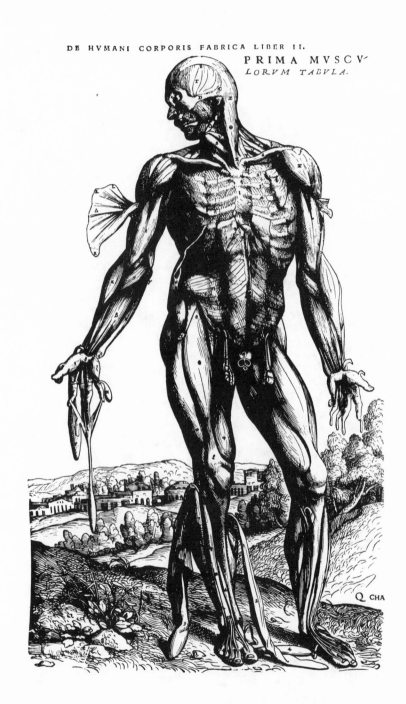

Q CHA

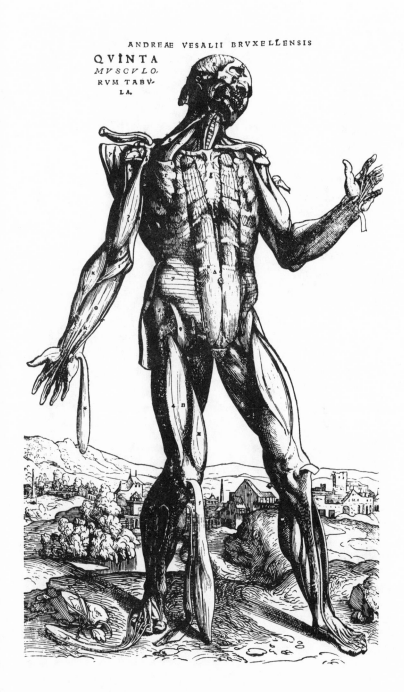

ANDREAE VESALII BRVXELLENSIS

QVINTA
MVSCVLO.
RVM TABV-
LA.

SEXTA
MVSCVLO-
RVM TA-
BVLA.

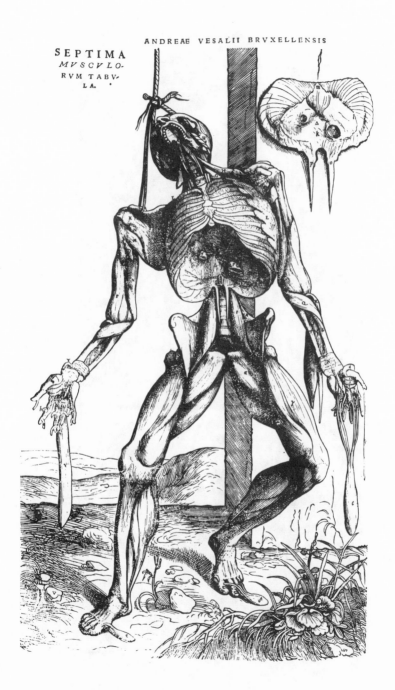

SEPTIMA
MVSCVLO-
RVM TABV-
LA.

ANDREAE VESALII BRVXELLENSIS

ANDREAE VESALII BRVXELLENSIS

OCTAVA
MVSCVL-
RVM TABVLA

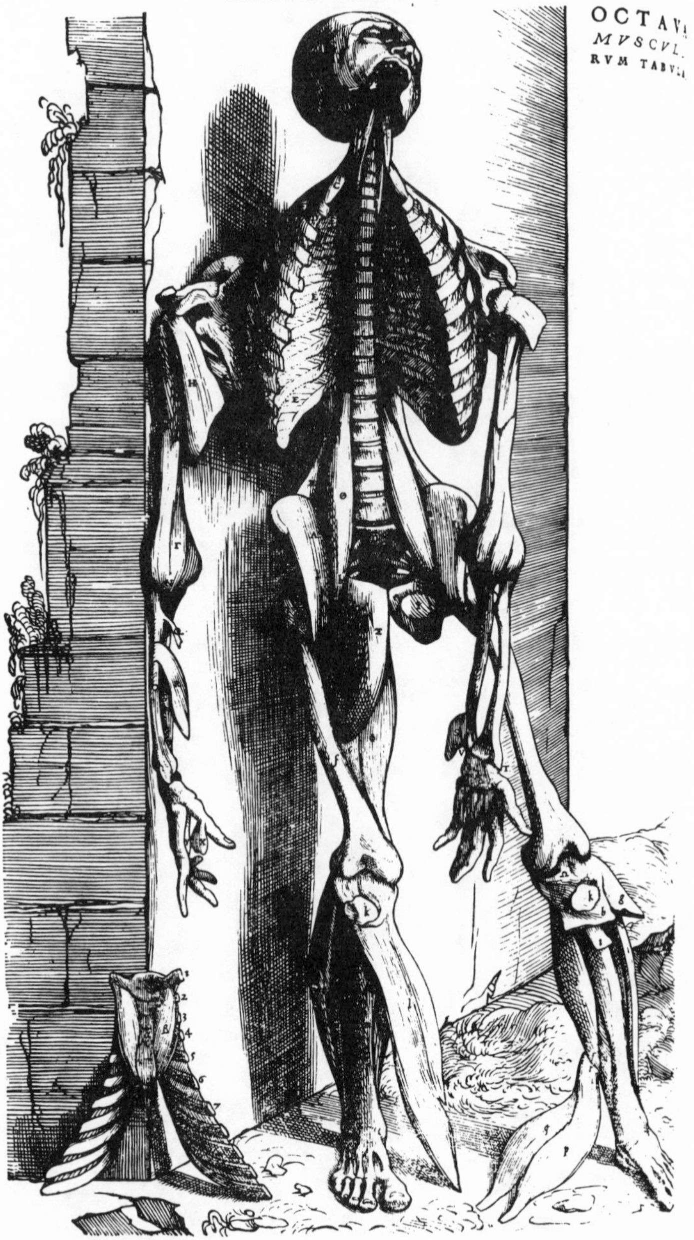

justify this violence is to give the body a negative emphasis—it is an idol or an absurdity.

The anatomist turns his process of negating forms into a positive program for revealing the truth by assuming the existence of a separation between false forms and true contents: by cutting away illusory forms or "idols," he will penetrate to the "real" truth. So, for example, Mainardo insists on the difference between empty forms of "Custom" and truth itself: "we ought to take hede not to Custom, not to the continuance of tyme, not to the multitude, nor to the authority of our elders, but to the only word of God, as Exechiel the prophet saith, walk not in the commandment of your father nor keep not there [sic] judgments, with there idols defyle not your selfs. . . ."[15] By placing the truth, "the only word of God," at a vast distance from man, and by discrediting the forms that might embody that word ("Custom," "multitude," "elders," "father"), Mainardo articulates a program for the anatomy that can never succeed. For the process of exposing idols does not lead to the revelation of an unsullied truth, "the only word of God." Instead, the procedure creates and discovers the world Donne describes in his "Anatomy" as "corrupt and mortal" in its "purest part."[16] The correspondence between microcosm and macrocosm is lost; matter no longer communicates transcendent meaning. The absolute decay of the world leads Stubbes's Philoponus to remark gloomily: "no man in anie catalogue, how prolixe soever, is able to comprehend the summe of all abuses their [sic] in practice."[17] The anatomist would like to insure the morality of the world but ends up confirming its essential materiality. In a brief survey of anatomies, Ronald Paulson remarks on the paradoxical relationship between the anatomist's pious goals and his technique for achieving them: "What makes these writers interesting after three hundred years is, in fact, the mass of detail with which they clutter their search for the absolute."[18] In other words, the anatomist's passionate effort to get back to a solid unified truth leads him to interrupt that totality and transform it into fragmented matter. But a significant change has occurred: the spiritual and the abstract are replaced by the sensible and the visible.

By representing his subject as a body to be dissected, a pious anatomist like Mainardo condemns vice to a worldly materiality and, at the same time, reveals his own preference for a language attached to visible matter. When Mainardo insists that "idols defyle" an invisible truth, "the only word of God," he sets up a hierarchy that privileges a nonmaterial truth over a sinful materiality. This is a familiar maneuver. Western tradition, as Derrida points out, has always elevated speech, spirit, the logos, over the exteriority of the body and the externality of artificial representation.[19] The process of anatomy itself challenges this hierarchy by putting the existence of a nonspatial truth into question: anatomy renders the invisible presence of the "word of God" into fragmented matter in order to make it visible. This visible matter becomes the objective truth of science, a truth still opposed to artificial forms of representation, "idols."

In anatomies, one class of idols is named "literature." Bacon, for example, claims that his philosophy is "true and severe (unencumbered with literature and book-learning)."[20] His hope to establish a nonliterary science might well have found encouragement in the discoveries of "spiritual" anatomists. They attempted to purify the body politic by dissecting the sins that beset it; yet in spite of their therapeutic intentions, this process of purification became a reductio ad absurdum that emptied out the traditional order and presented it as corrupt to the core. The discrepancy between customary, "literary" views of the world and the world made visible through anatomy makes clear why Bacon chose to adopt the process of anatomy for his writing: by exposing the idols of custom, by anatomizing the world as it is, men would make real progress in understanding. Progress, modernity, apparently lead men out of literature to experience and the world: Paul de Man has observed that advocates of modernity are often people who "stand outside literature."[21]

But though Bacon distances himself from literature through his stance as an objective scientist, even his efforts to cut away idols and discover the "real" lead him back to problems of language. Think of his efforts to bypass language by adopting an aphoristic style, for example. Unlike the suspect, wordy style of writing that Bacon calls "magistral," aphorisms are meant to present kernels of truth. Yet, as I will show in more detail later, these kernels are often more enigmatic than magisterial pronouncements. Even Bacon's most spare language, then, calls attention to itself as a medium that obscures the relation between words and things. What we can see here is how the paring away of a body turns the depths, the hidden truth, into matter not bound to an objective referent. Of course, if we sympathize with Bacon's desire for a knowledge of fundamentals, anatomy retains power as a necessary, if difficult, tool of investigation. But because anatomies are fond of rhetorical and visual displays— inevitable features of a method that turns bodies into parts, substance into surface—it is easy to suspect that anatomists are sometimes more concerned with showing off their technical skills than with revealing some elusive truth.[22] Certainly Lyly and Nashe intend their anatomies as vehicles of self-exposure.

The propensity of the anatomist to indulge in displays of his own virtuosity leads Northrop Frye to call the anatomy an "extroverted form."[23] Philip Stevick also remarks on the anatomist's delight in manipulating forms. Anatomies, he says, "tend to pursue abstract design, form for form's sake, to construct a rhythm of interruption, digression, and calculated inconsistency. . . ."[24] Ironically, an initial distrust of language leads finally to a vivid assertion of the domination of words over things. In a sense, anatomies are forms that have no reference— and that makes them into pure fictions, into radical forms of literature.[25] Literature provides both "scientific" and "spiritual" anatomies with a common home, or, perhaps, a common homelessness. But this way of talking about the space of anatomy does not immediately allow us to account for the energy and delight that anatomies display so enthusiastically. If the anatomy is destined to fold back on itself and discover only its own fragmented textuality, why do writers choose to repeat and repeat that motion?

My answer requires the assertion of more paradoxes. In the anatomy, the experience of the limits of form is a moment of departure as well as one of return. A knowledge of the constraints of form may engender a sense of imprisonment—recent criticism is all too full of such a feeling of loss and ending—but a sense of limits may also awaken a desire to cut through forms and grasp what exists beyond them.[26] That unknown region is present and yet absent in anatomies—it is the purity of an unfallen world that the anatomist would recover by stripping away false forms, or it is a nowhere of the future, a utopia that can be established if man finally penetrates to the essence of things and lives within truth and harmony. These totalities of past and future remain elusive because the anatomist's fragmenting method defers and distances the absolute order that he hopes to bring to light. For the anatomist, there is always more cutting to be done. The anatomy, then, is destined to face on a space beyond form that alternately fills the anatomist with the promise of a great discovery and a melancholy certainty of the world's decay.

Both responses are possible because the anatomist reveals a double dislocation of the truth—the traditional system of correspondences is exposed as corrupt and outmoded by a "science" that knows its own dependence on rhetoric. The anatomy, in other words, cuts both ways and thus raises an important question about both old and new styles of knowledge: How do we find the truth and restore the proper relation between words and things? The anatomy's concern with this epistemological problem reveals it as a transitional form, a form uncertain about its relation to an older discourse of patterning or to the new analytical discourse of science that it helps bring into being. Its allegiance, however, is to the new. This allegiance is shown in the "scientific" name—"anatomy"—that is adopted to describe the effort to reground knowledge through the act of separating appearances from reality. Even if the anatomy often ends up showing the hollowness rather than the substance of "reality," its transformative power may depend on severing meaning from form. Revelations of the hollowness of language encourage a liberating movement to expand knowledge and develop new styles of discourse. It is for this reason that the anatomy has an important role to play in the founding of our own powerful methods of analysis.

Certainly it is a passion for finding out the truth that gives intensity and breadth to the work of Shakespeare, Bacon, and Burton. And, as Nashe enthusiastically demonstrates, should the quest for truth fail, the anatomist can dismember the body in revenge. He may also, like the sophisticated Lyly, turn the loss of deep meanings into an opportunity to indulge in the sensuous surfaces of style, of external form. All the innovative anatomists I am concerned with offer compelling reasons for undertaking a study of the dissecting mode of composition. For the reader, there remains another lure: the hope that my method of writing will make visible the hidden structure of the form of anatomy. My study of anatomies has taught me how difficult it is to fulfill such hopes. So, in the following chapters, I am not going to place the form of anatomy on an operating table and expose its bare bones. Leonardo da Vinci, that great artist-anatomist, warns: "O painter skilled in anatomy, beware lest the undue prominence of bones and sinews and muscles cause you to become a wooden painter. . . ."[27] As important as bones and sinews and muscles, are ruptures and fissures filled with mysteries that cannot be easily formalized. Burton reminds the reader of his anatomy that its voice is elusive: "I would not willingly be known."[28] But by following the movement of the anatomy forward and away from the silent truths of bodies, by sharing the excitement of discovery and the melancholy of loss and decay, we will begin to see what it is to write anatomically.

2 · *Anatomy as Wit*

JOHN LYLY's *Euphues: The Anatomy of Wit* is one of those refined works too stylish to be meaningful and too deliberately artificial not to be. The superficial embellishments of such a work can be enjoyed the way Baudelaire enjoys the fashionable woman: "It matters very little that her ruse and artifice are recognized by everyone if their success is sure and the effect always irresistible." To those who claim that simplicity enhances beauty, he responds that this statement is equivalent to saying "that which does *not exist* enhances that which exists."[1] Undoubtedly the elegant Lyly would have applauded this aesthetic judgment because in his work, style is everything—it is both decoration and substance. Of all the Elizabethan anatomists, Lyly saw most clearly that anatomy is a method that produces a convergence of surface and substance. He sets out to anatomize wit because he wants to display it.

Yet this bright portrait of Lyly's anatomical endeavors is not quite accurate. The sexual metaphor employed by Baudelaire hints at a problem: to establish a work as feminine—and two well-known commentators on Lyly, J. Dover Wilson and R. Warwick Bond, attribute the success of *Euphues* and its sequel to their appeal to feminine sensibilities—has long been a way to point at weakness.[2] Because, as Lyly well knew, great authors are supposed to write works of substance and not of pretty surfaces, the relentlessly antithetical *Anatomy of Wit* has as one of its aims the separation of masculine virtue from feminine deceit. In fact, the anatomy so strongly attempts to divide masculine

substance and feminine surface that Bond describes passages of
Euphues as "misogynistic."[3] Lyly's book appeals to substance in
another way. He writes in order to court an audience that might
reward him with property and position (a place as Master of
the Revels was his particular goal). His witty productions did
not earn him this place and Lyly ultimately valued his achievement as nothing: to Elizabeth I he writes, "Thus Casting vpp:
an Inventorye of my ffrindes, hopes, promises, and Tymes, the;
Sum̄a, Totāl: Amounteth to Just nothinge. . . ."[4] As we will
see, Lyly's *Anatomy* reflects this judgment: it is a work of surface that critically exposes its own rhetorical condition. As G. K.
Hunter has argued, the work of John Lyly marks both the zenith
and the end of a humanist aesthetic based on highly formal
styles of patterning.[5] The method of anatomy has a role to play
in this paradoxical achievement of Lyly's playful wit.

The double-sidedness of Lyly's showy "anatomy" has long
bothered critics who want to place it once and for all in either
a rhetorical or a logical tradition. Is the *Anatomy of Wit* surface
or substance? But even one hundred years of debate have not led
to a conclusion about whether "euphuism" (the name Gabriel
Harvey gave to Lyly's style) is mere ornament or a technique of
analysis. Hunter sums up the irreducible ambiguity of Lyly's
style when he says that it "traces a line of scholastic logic which
is at the same time a line of rhetoric. . . ."[6] The same confusion of show and substance characterizes his subject—wit—and
his means of analyzing it—anatomy. Wit is both a faculty of
reason (an inward wisdom) and a talent for using words (an
outward facility).[7] And in his hands, anatomy becomes a technique that both creates and collapses the dichotomy between
rhetoric and logic, wit and wisdom.

Though the results of his technique are confusing, Lyly's
choice of the word "anatomy" to describe his work seems to
indicate that he wanted to conduct an analysis that would put
everything in its place. His conspicuous use of rhetorical conventions and his care in the construction of sentences and paragraphs reveal his intention to create an extensively ordered work.
A desire to distinguish things is also reflected in his use of
antithesis as the means of carrying out his anatomy. This focus
on contradiction, according to Jonas Barish, is the central differ-

ence between Lyly and his predecessors: "where his predecessors had aimed at exposing a hidden consistency in the workings of nature, Lyly arranged the affinities and antipathies side by side so as to unveil the contradictions in nature, the infinite inconsistency of the world."[8] In opposition to the harmony of microcosm and macrocosm, Lyly presents the world as an order divided against itself.

In the "Epistle Dedicatory" to *Euphues,* Lyly disclaims responsibility for presenting the world as a locus of disorder. An anatomy, he tells us, reveals only the objective truth:

> For as every Paynter that shadoweth a man in all parts, giveth every peece his iust proporcion, so he that disciphereth the qualities of the mynde, ought aswell to shew every humor in his kinde, as the other doth every part in his colour. The Surgion that maketh the Anatomy sheweth aswel the muscles in the heele, as the vaines of the hart. If then the first sight of Euphues, shal seeme to light to be read of the wise, or to foolish to be regarded of the learned, they ought not to impute it to the iniquitie of the author, but to the necessitie of the history.[9]

According to this testimony, the corpus of *Euphues* is a product of external necessity rather than artistic design. Lyly underlines the "necessitie" of his portrayal of *Euphues* later in the "Epistle" when he extols the virtue of tales that "set forth the naked truth" as opposed to those that clothe the truth in "finer speach than the language will allow" ("Epistle," 1:181). But since the extravagant finery of "euphuism" has made it a word that designates any ornate style of writing and speaking, Lyly's statements of his commitment to the "naked truth" seem playfully ironic. This most self-conscious of writers certainly knew that his style was a mannered one.

If we take the passage on anatomy to be playful rather than serious, we notice that in spite of his apparent concern with depth and objectivity, this concern is subverted by an opposed emphasis on the paintedness of the world revealed by an anatomy. Like the rest of the "Epistle," the passage is full of references to portraits, colors, the visible body of things, which suggests Lyly is merely playing with the scientist's claim to objective knowledge. In a letter "To the Gentlemen Readers" that follows, Lyly continues to assert the superficiality of his text by equating "Printers and Taylors," books and fashions: "a fashion is but a dayes wearing, and a booke but an howres reading, which seeing it is so, I am of a shoemakers mynde, who careth not so the shooe hold the plucking on, nor I, so my labours last the running over" ("Letter," 1:182). All this seems to indicate that Lyly, the writer who really inaugurates the form, is perhaps the one who best understood that an anatomy transforms a subject into an external display, a painting perhaps, of transitory and discontinuous matter.[10] More content with artifice than were those who followed in his mode, Lyly clearly expresses the fascination with matter that leads an anatomist to empty out the world and depict it in scenes, pictures, and images. In this respect, his anatomy is more witty show than substance, more concerned with masks than objective truths—perhaps because Lyly felt masks *were* the basis of reality.

But Lyly's love of the visible, a love that eventually led him to the drama, is tempered by the suspicion of surfaces that always inspires a writer to undertake an anatomy. The story of *Euphues,* is, after all, meant to teach the dangers that lie in a love of the external beauties of women and wit: "Euphues beginneth with love as allured by wit, but endeth not with lust as bereft of wisdome. He wooeth women provoked by youth, but weddeth not himself to wantonesse as pricked by pleasure" ("Epistle," 1:180). The instruction of Euphues and his readers depends on Lyly's ability to expose the difference between wit and wisdom. To do this, he creates polarities (wit and wisdom, love and lust) that seem to insure that positive values will be absolutely separated from negative ones. Yet Lyly's antithetical style not only creates a major polarity *between* wit and wisdom, it also creates positive and negative poles *within* each of these terms. In this way, the relentless use of antithesis subverts values: wit and wisdom are both good and bad, "For neyther is ther any thing, but yt hath his contraries" (*Euphues,* 1:196). Because the world of *Euphues* is morally ambiguous, its characters are constrained to use a discourse of equivocation. That discourse is "euphuism." It is not clear whether "euphuism" reflects the shifting values of Lyly's society or the inconstant nature of wit. One question to ask, then, is whether it is Lyly's witty style or his society that lacks a clear, decidable value system. The best way to get at an answer is through a close reading of *Euphues*.

When Euphues departs from Athens in order to travel to Naples, the dislocating process of the "anatomy" begins. The distance between Athens and Naples is moral and social as well as physical: Athens represents inward wit or "reason" and the institutional source of knowledge, the university; Naples, opposed to all that Athens stands for, represents the superficial language of "courting" and the sophisticated life of the city. This rigid opposition is immediately complicated in the opening dialogue between the young wit, Euphues, and the wise Eubulus who surprisingly defends the value of surfaces. Advising Euphues on how to avoid sin, Eubulus tells him that proper nurture, education by means of images of vice, enables men to do without the experience of vice itself:

> The Lacedemonians were wont to shewe their children dronken men and other wicked men, that by seeinge theire filth they might shunne the lyke faulte, and avoyde suche vices when they were at the lyke state. The Persians to make theire youth abhorre gluttonie woulde paint an Epicure sleeping with meate in his mouthe, & most horribly overladen with wine, that by the view of such monsterous sightes, they might eschewe the meanes of the like excesse. (*Euphues*, 1:188)

Ascham, in *The Scholemaster*, offers a powerful justification for an education based on a purely visual code: "Learning teacheth more in one yeare than experience in twentie: And learning teacheth safelie. When experience maketh mo miserable. . . ."[11] Here the voices of traditional wisdom, Eubulus and Ascham, endow surfaces, even tableaux of vice, with an elevating virtue while the substance of life is deplored as a dangerous enticement to corruption. Though both men occasionally argue against experience on the basis of their own experience, they most often insist that learning is best done by proxy, through the intervention of formal codes rather than in the world itself (a jus-

tification, no doubt, for a highly formal anatomy like Lyly's).
In this instance, Eubulus presents images of vice because antithesis determines that one thing leads to its opposite—vice to
virtue.

Euphues' response follows this law of contradiction. Eubulus
insists on the importance of nurture, so Euphues responds by
arguing the primacy of nature over nurture, experience over the
wisdom of "crabbed age." It is conventional that youth takes the
side of nature: by challenging the claim that the world is fully
explicated, fully codified in books and pictures, Euphues releases
for himself the possibility of discovering something new. Yet,
though he challenges the codes of the past, his arguments in
favor of nature are drawn from a store of proverbial doctrine.
Instead of escaping traditional wisdom, he exposes its contradictory nature from within. Euphues himself points out that
tradition provides him with arguments against tradition: "Now
whereas you seeme to love my nature, & loath my nurture, you
bewray your own weaknes, in thinking yt nature may any waies
be altered by education, & as you have ensamples to confirme
your pretence, so I have most evident and infallyble argumentes
to serve for my purpose . . ." (1:191). Between such firmly
established antithetical positions ("wee in all points contrary to
you, and ye in all points contrary to us") there is no possibility
of compromise. Euphues says as much to Eubulus: "Seeing therefore it is labour lost for mee to perswade you, and winde vaynely
wasted for you to exhort me, heere I founde you, and heere I
leave you, having neither bought nor solde with you, but
chaunged ware for ware . . ." (1:194). Through the operation
of antithesis, discourse has reached a dead end. By separating
positions so carefully, and by balancing them so evenly, Lyly's
method of dissection gives neither man the power to persuade
his opponent.

Though both Euphues and Eubulus are frustrated by the
exasperatingly binary structure of the text, Euphues' position
allows him to complain about the limitations of language. At
one point he tells Eubulus that language, like the old man, is
distant from life and action: "In my iudgement Eubulus, you
shal assone catch a Hare with a Taber, as you shal perswade
youth, with your aged & overworn eloquence, to such severitie

of lyfe, which as yet ther was never Stoycke so strict, nor Iesuite so supersticious, neyther Votarie so devout, but would rather allow it in words then follow it in workes, rather talke of it then try it" (1:193–94). His parting shot at Eubulus contrasts physical potency and linguistic power: "The Birde Taurus hath a great voyce, but a small body, the thunder a greate clappe, yet but a lyttle stone, the emptie vessell giveth a greater sownd, then the full barrell" (1:194). All this is consistent with Euphues' view that nature is a more powerful force than humanist codes— but, here again, he attacks from within "overworn eloquence." His critique of his opponent's style thus doubles back and undercuts his own.

The very language of the text, which is the same no matter what character is speaking, denies the possibility of a real difference between Euphues and Eubulus, wit and wisdom. This lack of real otherness, a lack that exists in spite of all the dividing and separating, breeds the distasteful narcissism of Euphues' character.[12] And it means that Euphues can never succeed in being the rebel we might want him to be. After he makes his attack on the codified order of wisdom, he immediately accepts the codified order of friendship: "I have red (saith he) and well I beleeve it, that a friend is in prosperitie a pleasure, a solace in adversitie, in griefe a comfort, in ioy a merrye companion, at all times an other I . . ." (1:197). For Euphues, relationships are possible only with another who is "the expresse Image of mine owne person." As Hunter and others have noted, Philautus, the name of his new friend, means "self-love." René Girard has described how desires are generated within relationships based on sameness: a man who is a mirror simply imitates the desires of others.[13] Lyly's text, frozen by antithesis, is able to move forward only because Euphues imitates his friend's love for a woman and, as a result, the story generates a new polarity—love and lust. The opposition of love and lust reverses the positions of surface and substance that were established in the first part of the story. Images, formerly lauded by wisdom, now become a source of vice; sexuality, once opposed to language, is now equated with it. This reversal of the values associated with show and substance makes it all the more difficult to tell where values lie—in surfaces, beneath them, nowhere?

The confusion about what is shadow and what is substance is dramatized when Philautus introduces Euphues to his fiancée as his "shadow." The "shadow" quickly proceeds to become the substance of Lucilla's love. Euphues' love for Lucilla comes from the outside, from Philautus, from Lucilla's beautiful form ("Euphues at first sight was so kindled with desyre . . ."), and Lucilla's love for Euphues originates in the exteriority of words, in Euphues' superficial wit. Euphues reveals his wit when entertaining the gathered company with proofs that a man ought to respect "inward qualities" more than "outward beauty": "Doe we not commonly see that in paynted pottes is hidden the deadlyest poyson? . . . Doth not experience teach us that in the most curious Sepulchre are enclosed rotten bones?" (1:202). Here Euphues is playing the part of an anatomist exposing the difference between external form and inner substance. But because his words are opposed to his "desyre," which privileges external form, the role of the anatomist is subtly undermined. This anatomy merely gives the appearance of wisdom—it is actually a play of wit.

The ease with which Euphues can adopt a pose and then exchange it for another, his virtuosity as a debater, is demonstrated when he allows Lucilla to determine the position he will take in answer to the question "whether man or woman be sonest allured, whether be most constant the male or the female" (1:203). Lucilla decides to take the view that women are inconstant so that Euphues will have to argue against it. To her delight, his sophisticated wit quickly frames an argument in praise of women which contradicts all that he has just said about them. Women, he now claims, are images of constancy: they are forms of totality, wholeness, not forms of deceit. The language of debate becomes an instrument of seduction when he talks in this vein—in "courting," the language of learning is used to flatter not to teach. Lucilla falls in love with his flattering picture of women; Euphues is so moved by his own words he is unable to continue speaking. Narcissism, the doubleness of their views of women, and the confusion of the language of learning (Athens) with the language of love (Naples) make it impossible for Lucilla and Euphues to tell if their love has been communicated and returned. It is not surprising that after these debates, they retire to ask themselves such questions as "canst thou fayne Euphues thy friend, whome by thyne owne wordes thou hast made thy foe?" (1:206). Given the inconstancy of their words, the confusion of show and substance, secure answers to these questions are impossible to find.

We can see by now that though antithesis provides an authoritative and obvious method of organization, it also frustrates the linear development of the narrative and its ethical goals. A characteristic passage from the love soliloquies shows both how antithesis controls Lyly's language and how it fragments meaning. In a world where reciprocity is prohibited by antithesis, soliloquy is the ideal form of communication. In a soliloquy, the self doubles and opposes itself. For an example, I choose a passage of the sort one critic believes is a key to the shift from a literature that emphasizes masculine deeds to one that expresses a feminine concern "with the very feelings and hearts of the lovers."[14] Here then is Lucilla considering the pros and cons of breaking her vows to Philautus in order to become the mistress of Euphues:

> Ah wretched wench Lucilla how are thou perplexed? what a doubtfull fight dost thou feele betwixt faith and fancie? hope & feare? conscience and concupiscence? O my Euphues, lyttle dost thou know the sodayne sorrow that I sustayne for thy sweete sake. Whose witte hath bewitched me, whose rare qualyties have deprived me of mine olde qualytie, whose courteous behaviour without curiositie, whose comely feature without fault, whose fyled speach without fraude, hath wrapped me in this misfortune. And canst thou Lucilla be so light of love in forsaking Philautus to flye to Euphues? Canst thou prefer a straunger before thy countryman? A starter before thy companion? Why Euphues doth perhappes desyre my love, but Philautus hath deserved it. Why Euphues feature is worthy as good as I, But Philautus his fayth is worthy a better. I but the latter love is moste fervent. I but the firste ought to be most faythfull. I but Euphues hath greater perfection. I but Philautus hath deeper affection. (1:205).

The "doubtfull fight" in Lucilla's mind begins with a series of questions that propose antithetical ways of interpreting her love for Euphues. Antithesis creates opposed sets of words, "faith and fancie" for example, and alliteration connects them so that opposed words sound similar. Lyly's use of other devices—isocolon (balancing clauses of equal length), and paromoion (balancing clauses with the same sound pattern)—also has the effect of neutralizing the difference between antitheses. It hardly seems that Lucilla's analysis will do her any good, but after the questions that open the paragraph comes a series of parallel phrases that either show the bad effects of Euphues' good qualities or assert those good qualities by negating the antithesis that lurks within them (for example, "feature without fault" or "fyled speach without fraude"). Those negative characteristics "fault" and "fraude" surface as aspects of Euphues' character in the questions that follow: Lucilla calls Euphues a "straunger" and a "starter." The character of a stranger is later elaborated by Philautus: "what truth can there be found in a travayler? what stay in a stranger? whose words and bodyes both watch but for a winde, whose feete are ever fleeting, whose fayth plighted on the shoare, is tourned to periurie when they hoiste saile" (1:222). A "starter" is also a wanderer and someone who deserts from a cause, an inconstant person. Euphues' inconstancy, however, is also Lucilla's—she proceeds to make more antithetical statements. The first two are compound sentences composed of a phrase beginning with "why" followed by one that opposes it, beginning with the word "but." The relationship between the two parts of the sentence is metonymical rather than purely antithetic, one statement is simply adjacent to another whose difference is assured by the conjunction "but." At the end of the paragraph, the opposing parts of the sentences become separated into a series of short phrases introduced by the words "I but." The process of Lucilla's mind thus anatomizes statements into smaller and smaller units of opposition.

By the end of her soliloquy, Lucilla is no closer to a resolution of the "doubtfull fight" than she was at the beginning. Apparently, the purpose of the passage was not to lead her to a truth, but to display Lyly's skill at debate. The value of argument as rhetoric lies in its form alone and the pleasure we feel in seeing it reproduced so skillfully. One wag has likened Lyly's verbal performance to the antics of a man who would undertake to hop on one leg from New York to Albany: "He would excite attention because he was able to hop so far, and not because he was the exponent of a praiseworthy method of locomotion."[15] For this reason, Morris Croll does not want to call Lyly's dichotomizing style "antithetical"—he does not want to make thinking into a somewhat ludicrous spectacle. To illustrate what a figure of thought should really look like, he gives an example from Bacon's essays, "revenge is a kind of wild justice," which he says reveals "new and striking relations between things."[16] But this is not an example of antithesis and he provides no counter-example from Lyly. Is "the measure of love is to have no measure" so different from what Bacon does? No.

In his article on Lyly's prose style, Barish opposes Croll by explaining that an anatomy, or any analysis conducted by means of antithesis, was a traditional technique of learning based on the premise that to know a thing was to know its opposite. Presumably then, antithesis was used in order to define the world and make judgments on the basis of those definitions. But clearly Lucilla's antithetical analysis does her no good—it presents her with equal and opposed choices without providing her with a basis for choosing one over another. Lucilla has not gotten any closer to making a decision by the end of the paragraph and the reader has no reason to suppose that the text will not remain forever locked in her endlessly decomposing soliloquy. Instead of laying bare a positive truth, antithesis leads to an impasse. If anything, "euphuism" questions both "ornamental" and "analytical" descriptions of antithesis. As Richard Helgerson has said: "despite its seeming eagerness to reassert the content of the humanist curriculum and to reemploy the humanist didactic method, *The Anatomy of Wit* covertly and perhaps unconsciously undermines both."[17]

Helgerson's judgment is a response to the doubleness of the role of wit in *Euphues.* Wit is both a dissecting tool and the means for creating a seductive but superficial representation of analysis. The erotic and manipulative side of wit is emphasized in the encounter between Lucilla and Euphues. Euphues seduces

Lucilla with his wit and Lucilla finally conquers the balanced oppositions of her soliloquy by asserting passion as its dominant content. The analytic is conquered by the erotic: "Let my father use what speaches he lyst, I will follow mine owne lust. Lust Lucilla, what sayst thou? No, no, mine owne love I should have sayd, for I am as farre from lust, as I am from reason, and as neere to love as I am to folly" (1:207). Her momentary insistence on the dominance of lust allows the story to move slightly forward before it is caught again in the forward and back movement of antithesis. Like this one, the moments of passion or withdrawal that allow Lyly's narrative to progress are minimal—balanced oppositions normally impede temporal development. Yet these moments, little dramas of metamorphosis such as Lucilla's conversion from love to lust, prefigure Lyly's career as a dramatist. The fascination of his plays lies in the fleeting encounters of opposites that absolutely shift the ground of reality, turning substance into shadow, reality into a dream. Lucilla's transformation is not so magical as the scenes of metamorphosis in the plays, but it does have the power to teach us that opposites are not so far apart—lust arises out of love, wit contains wisdom, wisdom is subverted by its own corrupting wit.

In an attempt to control the radical duplicity of the world of *Euphues,* Lyly tries to separate the inconstant from the constant through a sexual dichotomy—woman versus man. Woman incarnates deceit; she appears to be one thing and is actually the opposite. Euphues, who had called Lucilla a "Saint" and the "Expresse Image of Eternitie," finds she is changeable, beautiful but inconstant. Lucilla acknowledges her fickleness as a movement beyond her control: "fancie giveth no reason of his chaunge neither wil be controlled for any choice . . ." (1:238). In response to her rebuff, Euphues piously reminds Lucilla of the evils of feminine duplicity. Yet the inconstant Lucilla is more true than Euphues. She admits her waywardness while Euphues must be reminded of his: "whosoever iudgeth mee light in forsaking of you, may thincke thee as lewde in loving of me, for thou that thoughtest it lawfull to deceive thy friende, must take no scorne to be deceived of thy foe" (1:238). Though feminine inconstancy is apparently outside and opposed to male truthfulness, Lucilla reminds Euphues that inconstancy is actually situated within him.

Euphues deceives his friend through words. The gullible Philautus, believing words to be constant images, or in Lyly's words, thinking that "all be golde that glistered," is an easy mark for a witty man. By manipulating words Euphues betrays Philautus and further breaks down the dichotomy between the truthful language of Athens and the lascivious language of Naples—Philautus later remarks that Greeks are liars. Clearly both Euphues and Lucilla provoke a crisis of representation, a mistrust of images. In spite of this, Euphues believes in his own rectitude: to justify misleading Philautus, he asserts that Lucilla's perfection is an object worth lying for. She is truth: in her "the disposition of the mind followeth the composition of the body," a beautiful woman must be a "Saint." Such a faith in appearance leads men into a "fooles Paradise" (1:215). Only Lucilla is not seduced by the promise of absolute certainty; in her inconstancy she embodies the play of differences within the text, the equivocations of "euphuism" itself.

Euphues and Philautus find themselves in a "fooles Paradise" because they desire women and words to be constant. As Euphues later remarks: "I addicted myselfe wholy to the service of women, to spende my lyfe in the lappes of Ladyes, my lands in maintenance of braverie, my wit in the vanities of idle Sonnets. I have thought that women had bene as we men, that is true, faithfull, zealous, constant, but I perceive they be rather woe unto men, by their falsehood, gelousie, inconstancie" (1:241). To enable himself to set forth the real truth with masculine vigor and certainty, Euphues goes into exile. He separates himself from women and the world and embraces a kind of death-in-life: "As therefore I gave a farewell to Lucilla, a farewell to Naples, a farewell to woemen, so now doe I give a farewell to the worlde, meaning rather to macerate my selfe with melancholye then pine in follye, rather choosinge to dye in my studye amiddest my bookes, then to courte it in Italy, in the company of Ladyes" (1:242). To these farewells he eventually adds a farewell to dangerous words: "Farewell Rhetoricke, farewell Philosophie, farewell all learninge which is not spronge from the bowels of the holy Bible" (1:287). The Bible, though itself jammed with antithesis, parallels, and "euphuism" in various places, is designated a secure verbal ground of wisdom. Absolute renunciation in exchange for absolute truth, false surfaces for solid substances.

But there is a problem. Euphues keeps writing letters from his place of exile in order to share his new-found truth with others. And when he writes, Lyly's equivocal style undermines Euphues' sincerity. Is the voice of the "reformed" Euphues any different from the one that deceived Philautus? Is this newly discovered truth but a simulacrum of virtue, a "fooles Paradise"? Are his words, as Helgerson suggests, simply a sop to the conservative men in power who could help Lyly further his career at court?[18] These questions can be asked because Lyly's style, with its endless pro and contra, never allows us to feel that we are in the presence of a unified truth. As long as Euphues speaks in the text, he expresses its inconstancy of style.

Because antithesis breeds equivocations, the sexual opposition—virtuous man/deceitful woman—inevitably breaks down. The inconstancy of Lucilla spreads to Euphues and "euphuism" itself, giving the whole text of the *Anatomy of Wit* a "feminine" duplicity. Lyly's style has been accused of "corrupting the language"; it is "elegant" but too attached to "adornment."[19] Sidney criticizes such a style of writing in his *Defense of Poetry:* "Now, for the outside of it, which is words, or (as I may tearme it) Diction, it is even well worse [than writing that lacks *Energia*]: so is it that hony-flowing Matrone Eloquence, apparrelled, or rather disguised, in a Courtisanlike painted affectation. One time with so farre set words, they may seeme monsters, but must seeme straungers to anie poore Englishman. . . ."[20] Based on a similar criticism of "painted affectation" is Jonson's character Fastidious Briske, whose infatuation with women and wit makes him a comic butt. Fastidious, who as Bond observes is a parody of Lyly, is fascinated with apparel and its effects on reality: "Why, assure you signior, rich apparell has strange vertues: it makes him that hath it without meanes, esteemed for an excellent wit: he that enioyes it with means, puts the world in remembrance of his means: it helps the deformities of nature, and gives lustre to her beauties. . . ."[21] With this we have come back to Baudelaire and the charms of works that, like fashionable women, use artifice to enhance nature. But the charms of apparel are transitory—the words of Sidney and Jonson confirm Hunter's claim that Lyly's style was a "victim of fashion."[22] "Euphuism" was spurned by writers, much as Euphues spurned Lucilla, to establish the difference between their truthful words and "Courtisanlike painted" ones.

What critics of "euphuism" have not seen is that the opposition to a painted style begins within Lyly's own text. When Lyly writes, "I have ever thought so superstitiously of wit, that I fear I have committed Idolatry against wisdom," he says "I fear" because he mistrusts the glittering surface of wit. He opposes this surface through an anatomy, though at the same time he believes, with Eubulus and Ascham, that surfaces have the power to improve men. We might say, then, that his anatomy exposes the courtly code of humanism as both a fashion and a truth. This double perspective illuminates the unstable status of learning and writing at Elizabeth's court. As Colin Clout complains, there is at court

> No art of schoole, but Courtiers schoolery.
> For arts of schoole have there smalle countenance,
> Counted but toyes to busie ydle braines,
> And there professours find small maintenance. . . .[23]

Lyly spent his wit prodigally and got nothing in return. He closes one of his celebrated petitionary letters to Elizabeth with "a repentence that I have played the fool for so long, and yet live."[24] But perhaps the court did not reward him because it too was bankrupt. According to Lawrence Stone, the conspicuous expenditure of the English aristocracy was "disastrous to not a few noble fortunes, and harmful to the prestige of the peerage as a whole."[25] We began with a question about whether Lyly's style or his society lacked a stable foundation; apparently style, author, and society found themselves in a precarious position. In order to make themselves visible, all transformed their own substance and value into a flattering but ephemeral spectacle.

This process of emptying out contents in order to make them visible is the process of anatomy itself. The confusion of surface and substance that results is perfectly captured in Lyly's style, a style that is at once rhetorical and analytical. Because of its doubleness, Lyly's work can be situated both at the center and in the margins of his society. The exemplary Elizabethan writer, Lyly "crystallizes and synthesizes Elizabethan society's attitudes into literary form" but in the process reveals it to be only an exquisite fiction.[26] Through this double perspective, the shimmering *Anatomy of Wit* presents the limits and possibility of anatomy. Its possibility lies in its use as a method of "crystallizing," or, to use an anatomical metaphor, of exposing the basic structure of a courtly social code. It poses a limit to this process by showing how an anatomy creates and discovers the superficiality of its object, and of itself. The *Anatomy,* like wit, "woman," and the world, is suspended between substance and shadow. Its indeterminacy, thematized in the betrayals of Lucilla and Euphues, leaves open the question of the essential value of literature and courtly society.

In spite of Lyly's insights into the ambiguities of his method and his world, the *Anatomy* lacks intensity because it is too balanced, too equivocal. All Lyly's attempts to go beyond artifice are immediately undercut—his work expresses a sense of containment that is instantly met with a cynical denial of the possibility of escape. The most interesting anatomies that follow *Euphues* are not so complacent, nor perhaps so sophisticated; they express a passionate desire to cut through the confining skin of artifice in order to recover the fullness of history and nature. The rationale for these aggressive anatomies is simple: the artificial forms of culture must be negated if one is to confront the immense and intoxicating mysteries that lie beyond them. Nietzsche writes: "We negate and must negate because something in us wants to live and affirm—something that we perhaps do not know or see as yet."[27] This might be the motto of Thomas Nashe.

3 · Anatomy as Absurdity

THOUGH THOMAS NASHE imitated John Lyly by calling his first work an anatomy, his dissecting technique produced a text that bears little resemblance to *Euphues*. No one has ever flattered *The Anatomie of Absurditie* by calling it elegant, graceful, or beautiful: it is a ragbag of materials that most critics have either ignored or dismissed as a young man's folly.[1] But youthful inexperience does not explain Nashe's continued attachment to a fragmenting and fragmented style. As I see it, the disorder that characterizes his work is a sign of his permanent attraction to the strategy of anatomy—a technique of composition that is also a method of decomposition. Nashe sharpened the cutting edge of anatomy and cut through formal orders to explore an area of fiction located beyond *Euphues.*

Such exploration, as Jonathan Crewe remarks in a recent book, is dangerous: "in common with many of his peers" Nashe "must embrace the risks of rhetorical impropriety and linguistic innovation in order to pursue a career under the peculiar conditions of the 1590's."[2] For the educated and impoverished writer there were two strategies of survival: he—and I use the masculine pronoun advisedly—might produce decorous writing in the remote hope that it would be approved and rewarded by aristocratic patronage or he might make an even less hopeful ploy to attract readers of the developing commercial presses. Nashe made a compromise by adopting a familiar mode, the anatomy, and infusing it with unfamiliar violence—a strategy that attracted occasional patrons, occasional booksellers, and never enough money. In McKerrow's biography, phrases such as "want of funds" are a familiar refrain.[3] Without position or financial security, Nashe continually had to promote himself through his writing: anatomy provided a useful vehicle for both self-exposure and rhetorical experimentation.

It requires violence to escape constraining forms. Nashe justifies the violence of his anatomy by proclaiming the virtues of negation: he will expose absurdity "that each one at first sight may eschew it as infectious, to shewe it to the world that all men may shunne it" (*Anatomie*, 1:9).[4] He further insists on the morality of his decomposing method by adopting a "satirical disguise." The satirist and the scientific anatomist have much in common: both share a talent for demolishing bodies and a fascination with the raw materiality of objects. The difference between them (and what makes Nashe's work more satirical than scientific) is that the satirist believes the empirical world is essentially meaningless—it is absurd.

Though Nashe rails against it, this world of meaningless matter is really his element. As G. R. Hibbard points out, "Nashe had comparatively little to say," and it was for this reason that the anatomy suited him.[5] Operating on the principle that the best defense is a good offense, Nashe distracts attention from the lack of content in his own work by attacking other authors and books that have "comparatively little to say." The dissection of vacuous linguistic bodies has another advantage besides operating as a good defense: as Nashe exposes the superfluous matter of other texts, that superfluity fills up his work, *is* his work. As long as Nashe is attacking a textual body he can keep his writing going—so he persists. Throughout his career, perhaps most successfully in the "flyting" pamphlets, Nashe uses his talent for dismembering literature as a means of creating it.

Because literature is the prime target of his invective, Nashe's *Anatomie* is a kind of protocriticism. At the end of the "Preface to R. Green's 'Menaphon,'" he promotes it by saying: "It may be, my *Anatomie of Absurdities* may acquaint you ere long with my skill in surgery, wherein the diseases of Art more merrily discovered may make our maimed Poets put their blankes into the building of an Hospitall" ("Preface," 3:324). The hospital is doubtless another Bedlam and poets its foolish inmates. At the beginning of the *Anatomie* he repeats his intention to "runne through Authors of the absurder sort . . ." (*Anatomie,* 1:9). The absurder sort of authors write romance, invective, bad poetry, and pseudo-science. These texts share a lack of semantic content; they are literary forms whose only substance is insignificant lascivious matter. Such works are "absurd," a word that comes from the root *surdus* meaning deaf, inaudible, insufferable to the ear. (At one point Nashe tells Harvey, ". . . you *mute* forth phrases.")[6] Absurd literature means nothing and yet strikes the reader with the force of a physical object, it is "insufferable." The connection between abusing words, treating them as dumb objects, and physical abuse is one that Nashe himself makes by writing an "anatomy" and promising to "runne through Authors." Though he complains against this practice in the "Preface" saying, "It is a common practise now a dayes amongst a sort of shifting companions, that runne through every Art and thrive by none" ("Preface," 3:315), he too is an author of absurd, abusive literature.

The *Anatomie*'s critique of literary form begins with an attack on romances. This attack involves an invective against their duplicitous subjects, women: the sentiments are those of the "reformed" Euphues. According to Nashe, romances are filled with dangerously superfluous words:

> they sette before us nought but a confused masse of wordes without matter, a Chaos of sentences without any profitable sence, resembling drummes, which beeing emptie within sound big without. Were it that any Morrall of greater moment, might be fished out of their fabulous follie, leaving theyr words, we would cleave to their meaning, pretermitting their painted shewe, we woulde pry into their propounded sense, but when as lust is the tractate of so many leaves, and love passions the lavish dispence of so much paper, I must needes sende such idle wits to shrift to the vicar of S. Fooles who in steede of a worser may be such a Gothamists ghostly Father. (*Anatomie,* 1:10)

This indictment of literature that is mere "masse" that contains no "matter" echoes Euphues' attack on the "overworn eloquence" of Eubulus: "the emptie Vessell giveth a greater sownd, then the full barrell." With its obsessive use of antithesis and alliteration, it also has a "euphuistic" style. "Euphuism," as we have seen, confounds show and substance, and here too, "masse" and "matter" converge. But in spite of these similarities between the language of Lyly and Nashe, the harshly critical tone of the passage is oddly juxtaposed with the equivocations of "euphuism." In this first work, Nashe is still groping for a style that is unequivocally hostile to form, a style of formlessness.

He approaches such a mutilating style when he attacks Puritan anatomists who create debris as a result of their efforts to cleanse the world. Colloquialisms rupture the formal style of "euphuism" when Nashe furiously dissects these "men of furie":

> who make the Presse the dunghill whether they carry the muck of their mellancholicke imaginations pretending forsooth to anatomize abuses and stubbe up sin by the rootes, when as there waste paper beeing wel viewed, seemes fraught with nought els save dogge daies effects, who wrestling places of Scripture against pride, whoredome, covetousnes, gluttonie, and drunkennesse, extend their invectives so farre against the abuse, that almost the things remaines not whereof they admitte anie lawfull use. (*Anatomie,* 1:20)

What is the difference between anatomizing abuses and anatomizing absurdities? Stubbe's *Anatomy of Abuses,* which Nashe attacks here, was a Puritan's attempt to restore a theologically sound reality; Nashe, who tells us "It is not of my yeares nor studie to censure these mens foolerie more theologically," meant his *Anatomie* as a defense of humanism. But though their ends are different, their means are the same. Nashe conceals this similarity, however, by attacking those writers who, like himself, make "the Presse the dunghill." The same thing happens in the anti-Martinist tracts—Nashe, Lyly, and others attempt to out-Martin Martin. The danger of this strategy, as Richard Harvey and other Anglicans noticed, was that the cure had all the symptoms of the disease it was to heal. Defenses of tradition had begun to take part in its demolition. As Nashe himself observes, attacks on vice often "extend the invective so farre against the abuse" that nothing survives except debris. In the process of stripping away excess, the anatomist creates it. In the end, an anatomy makes the physical dominant over the abstract, the parts more important than any abstract unity. "Nowadays," Nashe writes "To the Gentleman students," "drosse" is "as valuable as gold" and "losse as wel-come as gaine" ("Preface," 3:314).

In a *Grammar of Motives,* Kenneth Burke describes how "debunking" techniques employed to reform the world become sanctions for a view that holds disorderly and contingent matter as the essential substance of human life. According to Burke, when an author assumes the existence of a hidden coherence, that absent unity becomes an invariable which the author feels can be dropped from his discussion. His argument then focuses only on the particulars of life in pejorative terms, they are "vices" and "absurdities." The result of this silence about universals and emphasis on a corrupt atomistic world is a picture of the world that argues against the existence of universals. Burke links the reductive debunking approach to the trope of metonomy: " 'metonomy' is a device of 'poetic realism'—but its partner, 'reduction' is a device of 'scientific realism'."[7] Scientists, like moral reformers, employ devices of reduction in an effort to achieve order. Burke does not mention that even scientists may not find a "real" order by reducing the world: reduction does not necessarily lead from one "assumed" order to the discovery of a new one. It may simply enact a transformation—Nashe's work, in any event, has the feel of a metamorphosis in process.

Though debunking techniques create a picture of the world as a sphere of chaos, Nashe argues against the validity of such a view by insisting that how the world is perceived reflects only the mental outlook of the perceiver. Writers of invective, he says, attack the world not because objective conditions are bad, but because they have "mellancholicke imaginations." Subject and object merge. This relativity of inside and outside means that Nashe too exposes himself in the act of exposing others. He half acknowledges this: the "pensiveness" that gave rise to his anatomy and his own proliferation of debris ("But what should I spende my ynke, waste my paper, stub my pen, in painting forth their ugly imperfections") make him an "accessorie to Absurditie."

Nashe's *Anatomie,* as literature that makes literature an object of dissection, is necessarily self-reflexive. Nashe separates himself from literature in order to anatomize it, yet he connects himself to his object by illuminating, through his dissections, the nature of his own literary text. We learn from him to pay attention to the artificiality of language. We learn that the anatomist reveals himself in revealing the world. And next, when he discusses the practice of writers who prey on other works of literature by tearing them "peecemeale wise," we learn that dissection is a mode of composition. Nashe exclaims with passion: "Good God, that those that never tasted of any thing save the excrements of Artes, whose thredde-bare knowledge beeing bought at the second hand, is spotted, blemished, and defaced, through translaters rigorous, rude dealing, should preferre their fluttered sutes before other mens glittering gorgious array . . ." (*Anatomie,* 1:20–21). Then Nashe gives us quotations from Latin texts that repeat his admonitions against borrowing from the ancients. Of the *Anatomie of Absurditie* McKerrow writes: "The whole book is evidently a patchwork of scraps from others, containing little, if any, original matter."[8] In spite of Nashe's claims of superiority, he inevitably repeats the strategies of the literature he contemptuously dissects. He too is one of the "Vultures" who "inveigh against no new vice, which heeretofore by the censures of the learned hath not beene sharply condemned, but teare that peecemeale wise, which long since by ancient wryters was wounded to the death, so that out of their forepassed paines, ariseth their Pamphlets, out of their volumes, theyr invectives" (*Anatomie,* 1:20). Feeding on the textual bodies of others, Nashe gains literary life.

To differentiate himself from those who account themselves "holier because they place praise in painting of other men's imperfections," Nashe attempts to demonstrate the affirmative power of his negating process. He rehabilitates anatomy by extolling the value of poetry. "But graunt the matter to be fabulous," he asks, "is it therfore frivolous?" (*Anatomie* 1:27). In words anticipating Bacon's discussion of fables as hieroglyphs, he writes that "the thinges that are most profitable, are shrouded under the Fables that are most obscure . . ." (1:26). Poetry is therefore profitable because it is "of a more hidden and divine kinde of Philosophy" (1:25). To get at the truths buried in literature, the reader must separate superficial "obscure" forms from solid virtuous contents. The method of anatomy, which does just that, apparently provides the means for getting at the essential truths of literature. At the end of the *Anatomie,* Nashe takes it upon himself to instruct students in his method. One eccentric critic (who wants to show that all Elizabethan writers are Francis Bacon) is dutifully impressed: "under a rude exterior Nashe is an artist of great refinement and, more than that, aspires to be a national instructor."[9] The comparison of Nashe and Bacon does not do much for Bacon, but it shows how seriously the moral purpose of anatomy can be taken. Nashe, just out of the university himself, aspired to be a "national instructor" because he knew only too well that "young men are not so much delighted with solide substances, as with painted shadowes, following rather those thinges which are goodly to the viewe then profitable to the use . . ." (1:46).

But Nashe's effort to expose the truth is unsuccessful. His insistence on the need to get beyond surfaces is a ruse that allows him to keep attacking surfaces rather than presenting positive norms. He does not so much reveal the value of poetry as confirm the impossibility of getting to it. He continues to criticize literature, and even expands his attack on superfluous matter to include an attack on men who eat and drink too much, and care more for "outward garments" than "inward vertue." Finally, after making a conventional recital of the virtues of brevity and coherence, the *Anatomie* concludes.

This conclusion is put into question by Nashe's own methods of composition. His anatomy cannot be brief because it never arrives at the truth it wants to expose; it cannot be coherent because it breaks down form. The inability of the anatomist to unveil kernels of meaning in poetry challenges the utility of literature—does it really contain "hidden divinity"? And it challenges the utility of anatomy. Nashe himself feels that acts of knowledge may be more disruptive than constructive: "he shall never enter into the reason of the trueth, who beginneth to be taught by discussing of doubts" (1:43). If skeptical investigations post-pone arriving at the truth, Nashe is destined to attack absurdity rather than reveal profitable contents. The last words of the *Anatomie* are a warning to the overcurious to contain their in-vestigations "least their knowledge way them downe into hell, when as the ignorant goe the direct way to heaven" (1:49). The only release from the weight of the meaningless matter of this world lies in the silence and oblivion of ignorance. Death, the most powerful agent for decomposing bodies, proves the ultimate absurdity of human efforts to compose a final truth.

In the *Anatomie,* then, Nashe must fail to compose a vision of order. McKerrow says of the work that its "author seems to have had no general plan in his mind. . . ."[10] At best, the *Anatomie* is a kind of list of the assorted writings Nashe dis-likes, or apparently dislikes, since once anatomized they resemble his own fragmented work. What the *Anatomie* tells us is that the attempt to go beyond form to the truth only leads to the creation of a form of formlessness in which words are like the detached pieces of a dissected body. In later works Nashe learned to enjoy the freedoms of this verbal terrain, though none of his contemporaries wanted to join him there. The freedoms, the liabilities, and the violence of a fragmenting method of com-position are best displayed in the texts of the "flyting" match between Nashe and Gabriel Harvey.

The bulk of Nashe's later writing is devoted to his quarrel with Harvey and provides additional evidence of his attachment to anatomy as a method of composition. The destructive energy of the "flyting" is generated by this mode of composition rather than by any extratextual "causes." The "causes" of the quarrel were actually two other texts which used dismemberment as a means of composition: in *A Quip for an Upstart Courtier,* Rob-ert Greene inadvertently attacked a dead man (John Harvey had died just before the text appeared) and later, after Greene died, Gabriel Harvey wrote a vengeful and scandalous exposé of the circumstances of Greene's death.[11] In a grisly way, the mutilation of these two dead men set the style of the "flyting," or at least provided an excuse for it. Harvey and Nashe achieved literary life by means of death.

As with *The Anatomie of Absurditie,* the "flyting" pamphlets have "comparatively little to say." In his article, "Issues and Motivations in the Nashe-Harvey Quarrel," David Perkins looks for intellectual issues underlying the quarrel and comes to this conclusion: "We can even doubt whether *any* really clear-cut and important intellectual issue exists at all in the dispute."[12] Because he can find no intellectual issues, Perkins focuses on personal motivations for the "flyting" match. He says that Nashe wrote for the sake of controversy because controversy could sell pamphlets, and points out that Nashe states his lack of interest in issues in *Strange News:* "Gabriel . . . write of what thou wilt . . . and I will confute it and answer it. Take truth's part, and I wil prove truth to be no truth, marching out of thy dung-voiding mouth" ("Four Letters," 1:305). For Nashe, then, the "flyting" is the occasion to display the nimbleness and infinite hostility of his wit. Harvey, on the other hand, writes to express the "contempt of a dedicated man for a writer who seemed to waste his potentialities in the pursuit of trifling ends."[13] But Harvey would not have engaged in the match if he had not relished argument for its own sake, so his contempt for the "common Pamfletters of London," however heartfelt, seems hypocritical.[14] As a result of his hypocrisy, Harvey was more vulnerable to attack than his opponent. Nashe was not claiming to be anything but superficial.

When he attacks Harvey, Nashe goes after Harvey's pretense to be a serious and profound writer. In *Strange News,* for example, Nashe promises to "unbowell the leane carcass of thy [Harvey's] book" to show it contains no true substance (*News,* 1:272). His dissection reveals that Harvey's writing is "all matter and no circumstance." As usual, this discovery allows Nashe to indulge his fascination for words torn out of context, words dislocated from their connotative meaning, while pretending this fragmented stuff is Harvey's creation not his own. Harvey saw exactly what was going on: "his only Art, & the vengeable drift of his whole cunning, to mangle my sentences, hack my arguments, chopp and change my phrases, wrinch my wordes, and hale every sillable most extremely; even to the disjoynting, and maiming of my whole meaning. O times: O pastimes: O monstrous knaverie."[15]

Harvey's insight, however, did not stop Nashe from mangling, hacking, chopping, and disjointing Harvey's texts. This is his preferred mode of operation. It allows him to demonstrate his skill at invective while disguising his complicity in perpetuating the absurdity he dissects. Perhaps all parodists are guilty of such duplicity—they imitate the texts they make ridiculous.

Though in the "flyting" texts Nashe is still dependent on the material provided by his victim, he no longer is constrained by a moral pose as he was in the *Anatomie*. His freedom from ethical limits enables him to create a remarkable decomposing fictional universe. The later works, like the earlier ones, are filled with second-hand material, organized haphazardly, and powered by an impulse to do physical violence. But unlike the earlier works, they have humor, élan, and a style that is pure "Nasherie."[16] Nashe achieved this style by allowing his language to explode through the fissure in traditional forms that Lyly had designated through his use of antithesis. "Nasherie" ruins traditional forms and releases an uncontainable destructive energy— "the fire of our wit is left, As our onely last refuge to warm us" ("Preface" to *Saffron-Walden*, 3:19).

Nashe's *Have with You to Saffron-Walden* is a good example of a text in which a new fictional order is composed through the process of decomposition. Unlike the earlier pamphlets in which Nashe randomly attacks one text after another, here he constructs a complete new work, a mock "Oration," from snippets of Harvey's writing. In addition to making the object of anatomy his own fiction, he also dramatizes, fictionalizes, his method of attack by creating five characters who take turns criticizing the "Oration." In this work Nashe shows that he is finally self-conscious about his technique of composition. The results look like this:

Bentiu: More Copie, more Copie, we leese a great deale of time for want of Text.

Imp: Apace, out with it; and let us nere stand pausing or looking about, since we are thus far onward.

Oration

But some had rayther be a Pol-cat with a stinking stirre, than a Muske-cat with gracious favour.

Bentiu: I smell him, I smell him: the wrongs that thou

hast offred him are so intollerable, as they would make a
Cat speake; therefore looke to it, Nashe, for with one Pol-
Cat perfume or another hee will poyson thee, if he be not
able to answere thee.

Carnead: Pol cat and Muske-cat? there wants but a Cat
a mountaine, and then there would be old scratching.

Bentiu: I, but not onely no ordinarie Cat, but a Muske-
cat, and not onely a Muske-cat, but a *Muske-cat with
gracious favour* (which sounds like a Princes stile *Dei
gratia*): not Tibault or Isegrim, Prince of Cattes, were ever
endowed with the like Title.

Respon: Since you can make so much of so little, you
shall have more of it. (*Saffron-Walden,* 3:50–51)

Because the characters (Senior Importuno, Grand Consiliadore,
Domino Bentivole, Don Carneades, and Piers Pennilesse, a "re-
spondent" much like Nashe) do not really have separate per-
sonalities, the language of the dialogue seems to proceed on its
own. The dialogic method, however, dramatizes the fight with
Harvey as an aggressive community sport. Nashe collapses the
pretensions of Harvey's veiled words, his "Princes stile," by
placing them in a colloquial discourse generated by his speakers.
He then displays his own linguistic virtuosity (he "can make so
much of so little") by tossing Harvey's words about until he has
exhausted their meaning. When he has reached a dead end, he
takes another piece of the "Oration" (More Copie, more Copie)
and repeats the process of emptying out the meaning of Harvey's
text, or rather, of exposing its meaninglessness. Because Nashe,
as Hibbard says, exhausts the possibilities of a particular situa-
tion, "and then moves on," there is no connection between one
sequence and the next.[17] Yet though his method of anatomy
proceeds by exhausting and fragmenting a textual body, Nashe
manages to recompose the fragments he creates through the
unity of the mock "Oration."

In the next section of the same "flyting" pamphlet, Nashe
creates another unified body to dissect. In this instance, he com-
poses a "Life" of Gabriel Harvey, a life he shows to be constituted of degeneration and corruption. This "Life" is further
fragmented by Nashe's fictional speakers who interrupt the

recitation of the "Life" to comment on the course of Harvey's ill-fated career. The narrator also is allowed to disrupt the text and play with its language. For example, a discussion of Richard Harvey veers into derisive play with his name:

> This is that *Dick* of whom *Kit Marloe* was wont to say that he was an asse, good for nothing but to preach of the Iron Age: Dialoguizing *Dicke, Io Paean Dicke, Synesian* and *Pierian Dick, Dick* the true *Brute* or *noble Troian,* or *Dick* that hath vowd to live and die in defence of *Brute,* and this our Iles first offspring from the *Troians, Dick* against baldnes, *Dick* against *Buchanan,* little and little witted *Dicke, Acquinas Dicke, Lipsian Dick,* heigh light a love *Dick.* . . . (*Saffron-Walden,* 3:85)

Nashe often attacks the identity of his opponents by playing with their names in this fashion. Gabriel, for example, becomes "Gorboduck Huddleduddle," "Gabriel Scurveies," "Gobin a grace a Hannikin," "Gregroies Huldreicke," "Ienkin Heyderry derry," to name but a few of his incarnations. To decompose a unified self signified by a proper name, Nashe disperses it into the endlessly shifting forms suggested by the mere matter of a name, its sound. Or, as in the passage in which Nashe plays with Dick's identity, he scatters his enemy into all the fictional poses he has adopted as an author. This is "Nasherie"—a style that calls attention to language as something to be enjoyed for its own sake, for its vitality and the willful violence it does to the pretensions of self and morality: "Take truthes part, and I will prove truth to be no truth. . . ."

This process of transforming meaning and self into fragmented matter cuts into Nashe's own identity and work since the text he anatomizes is a reflection of his own. Nashe seems unconscious of this in the *Anatomie of Absurditie,* but by the time he writes *Have with You to Saffron-Walden,* he is aware that he is being eroded by his decomposing methods of composition. His anatomy of others lacerates himself: dissection becomes a technique of self-annihilation. Is he so much his own enemy that he can actually take pleasure in verbal suicide? The answer appears to be that he is so much his own enemy that he and

Harvey are indistinguishable, he does not know whom he kills. Identification with Harvey thus both disintegrates him and provides him with a perfect substitute, one that protects him from a knowledge of his suicidal practices that might stifle his vigorous destructive energies.

Sometimes Nashe blames his readers for his self-destructive violence. His readers, for the most part other writers whose pamphlets were sold in St. Paul's Churchyard, are "like those . . . that kindle fire by rubbing two sticks one against another, so, to recreate and enkindle their decayed spirites, they care not how they set Harvey and mee on fire one against one another, or whet us on to consume ourselves" (*Saffron-Walden*, 3:30). More typically, he takes his readers into his confidence and directs his aggression to a fellow author. The displacement of violence is usually so effective that Nashe can really enjoy destruction and the power it gives his writing: the connection between the anatomy of a man's public identity and literal physical dissolution gives the writing the power of death. Nashe's writing has that consuming power: "If thou wilt have the Doctour for an Anatomie, thou shalt; doo but speake the word, and I am the man will deliver him to thee to be scotcht and carbonadoed: but in anie case speake quickly, for heere he lies at the last gaspe of surrendring all his credit and reputation" ("Epistle" to *Saffron-Walden*, 3:17). Intent on the mutilation of others, Nashe was oblivious to the harm he did himself.

Nashe's oblivion could not be promised to all the authors who decided to use the method of anatomy. Perhaps seeing how that method dispersed the anatomist, most writers chose not to repeat Nashe's fictional experiment. In a decomposing text, the writer reveals himself to be a displaced part of the body politic—verbal freedom dramatizes the lack of a coherent self and a solid meaning. This is what bothered Gabriel Harvey: "Howbeit amongst all the misfortunes, that ever happened unto me, I account it my greatest affliction, that I am constrained to busy my penne, without ground, or substance of discourse, meete for an active and industrious world."[18] The nothingness both Harvey and Nashe discover at the bottom of all they write about is a mirror of the negligible position of writing and writers in Elizabethan society.

The position of that society was also insecure. The quarrel between Nashe and Harvey was ended by proclamation because it too keenly reflected the dangers of rebellion and the uncertainty of the future that haunted Elizabethan society at the end of the century. The order of censorship states "that all Nasshes bookes and Doctor Harveys bookes be taken where soever they maye be found and that none of their bookes be printed hereafter."[19] The order may be an admission that the anatomy was a subversive form of representation that, by negating fictions of totality, communicated the primacy of disorder and chaos. In a way, both Nashe and Harvey were Levellers. But Nashe, because he did not share Harvey's desire to put language in the service of statecraft, was, in spite of his conservative beliefs, the more dangerously destructive of the two.

Nashe's style, reducing the bodies of man and language into fragmented matter, respects no order at all. His leveling, debunking technique was a process of decay—but, more important to Nashe, it broke a path to a language freed from its old moral and rhetorical associations. When he enters into this language, Nashe becomes invulnerable to the attacks of his opponents because it is a language beyond self and judgment: "Holla, holla, holla, *flurt, fling,* what reasty Rhetoricke have we here? certes, certes, brother *hoddy doddy,* your penne is a coult by a cockes body" ("Four Letters," 1:281). The words are an end in themselves. By anatomizing form, Nashe revealed the absurdity of language and released its raw, insufferable energy. Shakespeare, a writer also willing to venture to the extremes of his medium, had to struggle with the reckless capacity of language to free itself from the imposition of any order.

4 · *Anatomy as Comedy*

AS YOU LIKE IT is a play constituted out of conflicting desires: the desire to escape the orders of language and society and the desire to celebrate them. It begins with an assertion of social and linguistic freedom against a repressive order, a movement of liberation or escape that C. L. Barber says is basic to the comic formula of "release to clarification."[1] "Release" is necessary because linguistic conventions constrain the creative energies of the lover and the poet; the patriarchal order represses women and youngest sons. But though Barber's formula implies that "clarification" is a consequence of "release," in *As You Like It* "release" seems to impede the construction of a comic unity. The subversive dynamic of "release," which opens up forms, also leaves the lovers unable to formalize their love in speech and marriage. At the end of the play, order is imposed on the emancipated characters in Arden to make this formalization possible—though even this happily clarified order cannot entirely satisfy the desire to reveal the "real" or "natural" that lies beyond form. Not everyone accepts a place in the comic order, some characters remain "out of doors," wandering in Arden, searching for something external to all man-made orders.

The mechanism of release in this play, of breaking through forms, is the method of anatomy. Shakespeare certainly had an "anatomy" in mind when he wrote *As You Like It:* the narrative source of the play is Thomas Lodge's "Rosalynde," subtitled "Euphues golden legacie: found after his death in his cell at Silexdra."[2] The legacy is the antithetical style of Lyly's *Euphues:*

The Anatomy of Wit, which Lodge adopted. His "euphuistic" narrative was produced by turning Lyly's anatomy inside-out: in "Rosalynde," friendship is true and not feigning, "country amours" are opposed to "courtly fancies," and women and men are as good as they appear to be. This process of reversal turns Lyly's antiromantic anatomy into a romance. Yet a necessary discord underlies the harmonies of "Rosalynde" because Lodge uses Lyly's technique of antithesis to create his picture of unity. Lodge himself acknowledges the aggressiveness of his romance in a "Letter to Gentlemen Readers": "Heere you may perhaps find some leaves of Venus mirtle, but heawen down by a souldier with his curtleaxe, not bought with the allurement of a filed tongue." The comic unity of "Rosalynde" bears the marks of a soldierly art—the marriage ceremony at its end is interrupted by a command that the men turn their "loves into lances."[3] In *As You Like It,* Shakespeare explores Lodge's anatomizing method of achieving order, a method of unification that requires the interruption of order.

A separation of the symbolic order from the plenitudes of truth and nature motivates any anatomy: there is no need to go beyond public forms to find a locus of meaning if forms are perceived as adequate representations of reality. In *As You Like It,* an attack on form is necessary because the realm ruled by Duke Ferdinand is inauthentic and unnatural. The duke has violated a fundamental law of feudal society, the law of primogeniture, by usurping the position of his older brother; Orlando and Adam tell us that "the service of the antique world" has been forgotten; and even the duke himself criticizes Oliver, Orlando's brother, for neglecting his familial obligations, the ancestral bonds that are the source of legitimacy for an aristocratic family. Of course the duke's reason for upholding the standards of propriety is mercenary—he punishes Oliver by sending him "out of doors" and claims his house and lands—yet his mercenary actions make the point again that the public realm has become divorced from its moral foundations.

When forms appear to lack essential value, they point to a significance that lies outside them, silent and good. The people silenced in Duke Ferdinand's realm stand for all his realm is not. Orlando, for example, represents an archaic ethical order, "the spirit" of his father. In an opening speech, he rebels against a brother who excludes him from the public sphere: "The courtesy of nations allows you my better in that you are the first born, but the same tradition takes not away my blood were there twenty brothers betwixt us" (I.i.42–45).[4] Blood, the body itself, challenges the public order in words that strangely prefigure Edmund's:

> Wherefore should I
> Stand in the plague of custom, and permit
> The curiosity of nations to deprive me,
> For that I am some twelve or fourteen moonshines
> Lag of a brother?[5]

But Orlando's rebellion against his older brother, which parallels Duke Ferdinand's rebellion against the good Duke Senior, does not seem sinister because nature (blood, the forest of Arden) is the site of value in this play. Orlando is noble by nature ("he's gentle, never schooled and yet learned") but as a youngest son he has no position in society ("Only in this world I fill up a place"). And Rosalind is in an identical position. As the daughter of the legitimate duke she is truly noble, but as a young woman without family she has no place in society. She, like Orlando, has nothing except the power to signify what society excludes. They both exist in a negative relation to the symbolic order.

Duke Ferdinand articulates Rosalind's power to signify what has been banished from the public order. It is not what Rosalind says, but what she does not say, what she cannot say given the limits of what can be spoken, that is dangerous to his realm:

> Thus do all traitors.
> If their purgation did consist in words,
> They are innocent as grace itself.
> Let it suffice thee that I trust thee not.
> (I.iii.48–51)

Rosalind threatens his control over the symbolic order by indicating meanings he wants to censor. Her words are innocent— but her silence, filled with what cannot be said, is subversive:

Rosalind's "very silence and her patience, / Speak to the people" (I.iii. 74–75). By banishing her, Duke Ferdinand hopes to make his order manageable, to make it seem complete and legitimate.

What is banished by Duke Ferdinand finds a home in Arden. The inhabitants of the forest break through appearances, they reveal occluded matter—in other words, they conduct an anatomy of order to bring hidden contents to the surface. Arden is a kind of antiworld, a place where all that is repressed in the "working-day world" can be figured forth. In this world turned inside-out, women appear to be men, men busy themselves with idle love, and language has the freedom to speak everything and nothing. The symbolic order is renewed, filled with power by an explosion of language and of love. These two mysterious entities lack a stable identity—they are playful, changeable, excessive. In this, they resemble the inhabitants of Arden who are wandering, transforming, displaced from home. Men and women, love and language, all participate in the dizzying freedom of Arden.

The disorienting center of the play, though it allows no one a secure place or identity, is a place of happiness because love is one of the things that is located beyond all order. True love "cannot be sounded," cannot be contained in a word or definition. Rosalind insists that attempts to formalize love are unnatural, as do Celia, Touchstone, and Jaques, in criticisms of Orlando's love poetry. His verses mar the trees they hang on, they reduce Rosalind to segments ("Helen's cheek, but not her heart, / Cleopatra's majesty, / Atalanta's better part . . ." [III.ii. 139–41]), and they quench the fire of love in banal formulas: "what tedious homily of love have you wearied your parishioners withal and never cried 'Have patience, good people!'" (III.ii. 149–51). The artifice of love falsifies its nature, makes love and the lover seem lifeless stereotypes—Jaques easily labels Orlando, he is "Signior Love." To release Orlando from convention, Rosalind "cures" him of love by leading him to its unorderable depths.

Her method of getting to those depths is an anatomy. As she explains to Orlando, her "cure" is a process of exposing and exacerbating her subject's disorder:

He was to imagine me his love, his mistress; and I set him every day to woo me. At which time would I, being but a moonish youth, grieve, be effeminate, changeable, longing and liking, proud, fantastical, apish, shallow, inconstant, full of tears, full of smiles; for every passion something and for no passion truly anything, as boys and women are for the most part cattle of this color; would now like him, now loathe him; then entertain him, then foreswear him; now weep for him, then spit at him; that I drave my suitor from his mad humor of love to a living humor of madness, which was, to forswear the full stream of the world and to live in a nook merely monastic. (III.ii.382–94)

The danger of her technique of teaching Orlando about love is that the portrayal of love's disorder can lead to the lover's separation from the orders of reason (a "living humor of madness") and society (life in a "nook merely monastic"). Fortunately, Orlando "would not be cured," for Rosalind's success would frustrate her desire for union. There is a risk involved in teaching Orlando the difference between love and false representations of it, just as there are dangers in a blindness to this difference, in Orlando's refusal to be cured.

Without Rosalind's lessons, Orlando could remain, like the shallow Phebe, infatuated with words when love is what escapes them. A love that defies all orders expresses itself only as endless contradiction:

I will be more jealous of thee than a Barbary cock-pigeon over his hen, more clamorous than a parrot against rain, more newfangled than an ape, more giddy in my desires than a monkey. I will weep for nothing, like Diana in the fountain, and I will do that when you are disposed to be merry; I will laugh like a hyen, and that when thou art inclined to sleep. (IV.i.136–42)

Here antithesis is a means of "release." When Rosalind puts on a mask, she does so to teach Orlando not to condemn her to one. She defines her "woman's wit" as an uncontainable energy: "Make the doors upon a woman's wit, and it will out at the casement; shut that, and 'twill out at the keyhole; stop that, 'twill fly with the smoke out at the chimney" (IV.i.148–51). Hers is an anatomizing wit, a wit that undermines forms. Rosalind adopts a role to subvert all roles, and displays her wit to announce that it is pledged to nothing. She tells Orlando that Rosalind has no consistent identity and so will appear to him in many forms, as an actress in many roles. In her demand for love's freedom and her own, she resembles Cleopatra—and also the skeptical Jaques.

As the comparison with Jaques indicates, Rosalind's radical doubt about the value of formalizing love could leave her, as well as her lover, in melancholy solitude. Love that is not communicated does not lead to the exchange of love that is basic to the union of lovers. When Rosalind sees that the debunking of roles and conventions has become an obstacle rather than a means to achieve her goal of marriage, she wearies of questioning and testing forms. The conflict between the indefinable nature of love and her desire to express it becomes apparent when she finds herself the only one of the lovers who cannot speak her love. The long passage in which Rosalind discovers herself caught between speech and silence deserves to be quoted in full:

Phebe:	Good shepherd, tell this youth what 'tis to love.
Silvius:	It is to be all made of sighs and tears;
	And so am I for Phebe.
Phebe:	And I for Ganymede.
Orlando:	And I for Rosalind.
Rosalind:	And I for no woman.
Silvius:	It is to be all made of faith and service;
	And so am I for Phebe.
Phebe:	And I for Ganymede.
Orlando:	And I for Rosalind.
Rosalind:	And I for no woman.
Silvius:	It is to be all made of fantasy,
	All made of passion, all made of wishes,
	All adoration, duty, and observance,
	All humbleness, all patience, and impatience,
	All purity, all trial, all observance;
	And so am I for Phebe.
Phebe:	And so am I for Ganymede.
Orlando:	And so am I for Rosalind.
Rosalind:	And so am I for no woman.
Phebe:	If this be so, why blame you me to love you?

Silvius: If this be so, why blame you me to love you?
Orlando: If this be so, why blame you me to love you?
Rosalind: Why do you speak too, 'Why blame you me to love you?'
Orlando: To her that is not here, nor doth not hear.
Rosalind: Pray you, no more of this; 'tis like the howling of Irish wolves against the moon. (V.ii.78–104)

Rosalind's love, because it eschews form, is absent, "not here." Orlando says it "doth not hear" because it does not respond to his entreaties. To make itself present, love must use artifice, must repeat and repeat time-honored sentiments. If it remains silent, and true to its own inexpressibility, love can only announce itself by saying what it is not: Rosalind says her love is "for no woman." But isn't such a negative relation to form more attractive than the conventionality of the others? The discourse perpetuated by Orlando, Phebe, and Silvius turns love into a "howling," into a frenzy of words that can speak love, but only by announcing a love (a conditional one, "if this be so") separated from its object: "Why blame you me to love you?" Rosalind cannot speak her love; Orlando can speak his love only to announce his utter separation from Rosalind. Between the lovers stand a disguise, words, representation. Yet what stands between them also links them, allows them to be coupled. It is that alienating realm of speech that gives love form and places it in the symbolic order where marriages take place. In the end, Rosalind decides to rein in her anatomizing wit, accept a role as reality, and reassert the primacy of public forms of order. She does this by embracing conventions rather than by demystifying them. All is accomplished with the help of an "if," Touchstone's peacemaker. This "if" is an ironic, though useful, maker of order, and with it Rosalind can magically make forms but she cannot consecrate them. Hymen must be brought in to transfigure the new order because Rosalind's wayward wit puts it too much in question.

Rosalind's wit makes wandering and disruption an end rather than a means to an end. It is opposed to permanence, to closure, on the grounds that "the wiser the waywarder" (IV.i.148). The association of her linguistic powers with magic is one sign of their uncanny and disorderly nature: in telling Orlando that her magic is "not damnable," Rosalind only reminds us that magic is diabolic and unlawful. Her mentor, "an old religious uncle" who "taught [her] how to speak" (III.ii.325–26) lives apart from society and from the laws that govern it. If Rosalind is in possession of his lawless and wonderful powers, she is also possessed by them. Word magic is hard to control—once the boundaries between illusion and reality have been blurred, it is hard to reestablish them.

In *Euphues,* John Lyly makes wit his field of research. He dissects "wit." At one point in the narrative he offers a commentary on the disruptive nature of his subject:

> Heere ye may beholde gentlemen, how lewdly wit standeth in his owne lyght, howe he deemeth no pennye good silver but his owne, preferring the blossome before the fruite, the budde before the flower, the greene blade before the ripe eare of corne, his owne witte before all mens wisedomes. Neyther is that geason, seeing for the most parte it is proper to all those of sharpe capacitie to esteeme of themselves, as most proper: if one bee harde in conceiving, they pronounce him a dowlte, if given to study, they proclayme him a duns, if merrye a iester, if sadde a Sainct, if full of wordes, a sotte, if without speach, a Cypher, if one argue with them boldly, then is he impudent, if coldely an innocent, if there be reasoning of divinitie, they cry *Quae supra nos nihil ad nos,* if of humanitie, *Sententias loquitur carnifex.*[6]

A wit, according to Lyly, is lewd, narcissistic, impatient, rebellious, and contrary. Lyly's own witty language is excessive, antithetical, and through its insistent use of the conditional "if," guarded against endorsing a truth. Rosalind's wit is equally "wayward," lewdly inconstant. In a demonstration of her wit, Rosalind tells Orlando she will have him and twenty other men as well, for "can one desire too much of a good thing?" (IV.i. 110–11). Here words lead her beyond the bounds of propriety.

A language "out of all hooping," a lover's language, is always "either too much at once, or none at all" (III.ii.192). Celia tells Rosalind, "Cry 'holla' to thy tongue, I prithee; it curvets unseasonably" (III.ii.232–33). Intoxicated by love, Rosalind has been overcome by language: she is in danger of enjoying her wit more than Orlando. As Roland Barthes says in *A Lover's Discourse,* "The fulfilled lover has no need to write, to transmit, to reproduce."[7] As long as Rosalind is not fulfilled, she can demonstrate her magic by creating substitutes for Orlando—words, fictions, illusions. In getting pleasure this way, Rosalind reveals that wit has become an object of desire, not a means to reach someone else: wit "deemeth no pennye good silver but his owne." Erotic and licentious verbal encounters thus usurp the place of marriage and human reproduction. The freedoms of wordplay, however, offer pleasures that are not of the body. Orlando finally tells Ganymede, "I can live no longer by thinking" (V.ii.48). Rosalind replies: "I will weary you then no longer with idle talking" (V.ii.49–50). She stops the production of verbal substitutes by the same means that maintained it—magic. With another sleight of hand, order will appear. How can we trust that this is the real thing, not an illusion? Having waylaid order with her magical wit, Rosalind cannot successfully redeem it. Shakespeare must bring in a god, Hymen, to compel our belief in the solidity of the order established at the end of the play.

The masque is a traditional form for resolving contradictions and paradoxes.[8] Shakespeare uses it to transform the stage into a vision of order: verbal design is sanctioned by a transcendent authority and the fecundity of nature is captured in the social form of marriage. Hymen announces somewhat abruptly:

Peace ho! I bar confusion:
'Tis I must make conclusion
   Of these most strange events.
Here's eight that must take hands
To join in Hymen's bands,
   If truth holds true contents.
(V.iv.119–24)

Hymen's "if" is unexpected and unsettling—it begins to decompose the order that has just been consecrated. His "if" causes a fissure between the form of truth and its contents that raises a question about the truthfulness of what appears true. Even without that subversive "if" there remains a tautology, one of the "vices of language."[9] In this instance, the tautology is an image of truth's inability to be other than itself, though ironically this image is logically false. Truth cannot be spoken truly because language is made up of signs that substitute for truth itself.

The celebration of the masque requires that all the participants give up their critical distance from external form and submit themselves to one in order to renew it. Enveloped in form, the celebrants lose their wit and their freedom, and the power to order passes from Hymen to Jaques, who is separate from the form of the masque. At this moment we are distanced from the structure of comic unity and forced to recognize that it is not inclusive—Jaques remains outside this supposed order created by an "if." Duke Senior beseeches him, "Stay, Jaques, stay." Jaques replies, "To see no pastime I" (V.iv.188–89).

By calling the celebration of marriage a "pastime" Jaques turns the comic resolution into a fiction, a form separate from serious truths that are to be found outside it. Throughout the play, he relentlessly attempts to negate forms—not to get at the truths of the body but to get at meanings uncorrupted by their physical casing. He is always searching for these pure and profound truths—Jaques remains in the forest to discover "matter to be heard and learned"—because he finds no body, no order that is a site of uncorrupted value. The inevitable contamination of worldly form provokes a desire for absolute "release." This radical form of "release" cannot be achieved so long as men are masked on the stage of the world or encased in the decaying flesh of the body.

Jaques is not the only one who questions the value of theatrical gestures of opening and discovering. Even in an early scene of the play, when "release" promises to take Orlando and Rosalind from "banishment to liberty," Oliver's attempts to reveal the hidden truth of Orlando put the efficacy of opening up forms into question. Denying responsibility for a self-serving exposé of his brother, Oliver says: "I speak but brotherly of him, but should I anatomize him to thee as he is, I must blush and weep, and thou must look pale and wonder" (I.i.143–45). His words reveal the theatrics of the anatomist, the anatomist's disgust at corruption, but nothing of the subject he desires to dismember. His anatomy, then, is not a technique of discovery but a technique of displacement. It is a circuitous method—by exposing others the anatomist exposes himself. When Jaques insists that "the wise man's folly is anatomized / Even by the squand'ring glances of the fool," Duke Senior responds:

Most mischievous foul sin, in chiding sin.
For thou thyself hast been a libertine,
As sensual as the brutish sting itself;
And all th' embossed sores and headed evils
That thou with license of free foot hast caught,
Wouldst thou disgorge into the general world.
(II.vii.64–69)

In this passage, the duke points out how the process of exposing others reveals the anatomist. Instead of getting at reality, at the nature of things, the anatomist covers up the world with images of himself, with the debris of his own corrupt life.

Depicted in this way, anatomy is not a positive method for bringing the truth to light, but a mechanism of self-exposure. Arden is haunted by the possibility that there is no way to go beyond self to another, beyond forms to nature. Both Phebe and Orlando are in love with mirrors of themselves: Orlando learns to love Rosalind by courting another boy; Phebe loves her own femininity which is reflected in Ganymede's.[10] Such narcissistic love, born of a process that discovers the self in others, impedes love-in-marriage, the familiar ritual of comic resolution: Orlando cannot marry another boy, nor Phebe another woman. Fortunately Rosalind is both a mirror and something else—she is self and other. But these categories, of course, are quite unstable and the play between them encourages the kind of confusion that Rosalind must resolve.

Jaques's defense of his negating technique, for example, depends on a denial of the difference between self and other. He tells the duke that whether he reveals himself or others, the result is the same, he exposes the endless vanity of men. All men narcissistically promote themselves until their energy for self-dramatization, the energy of life itself, is exhausted:

Why, who cries out on pride
That can therein tax any private party?
Doth it not flow as hugely as the sea
Till that the weary very means do ebb?
(II.vii.70–73)

To cure men of their folly, Jaques must "through and through cleanse the foul body of th' infected world" (II.vii.59–60). This cleansing will negate all the bodies of the world, reduce them to rubble, in an effort to return the world to order. The world, it seems, must be dismantled to be restored.

Jaques's melancholy is a reflection of such a fragmented world without a coherent meaning. This melancholy, like Rosalind's love, is better defined by what it is not than by what it is:

I have neither the scholar's melancholy, which is emulation; nor the musician's, which is fantastical; nor the courtier's, which is proud; nor the soldier's, which is ambitious; nor the lawyer's, which is politic; nor the lady's, which is nice; nor the lover's, which is all these: but it is a melancholy of mine own, compounded of many simples, extracted from many objects, and indeed the sundry contemplation of my travels, which, by often rumination, wraps me in a most humorous sadness. (IV.i.10–18)

This description provokes Rosalind's antivoyaging remark: "I had rather have a fool to make me merry than experience to make me sad: and to travel for it too" (IV.i.24–26). But Touchstone, the fool, has a brain in much the same state: "And in his brain, / Which is as dry as the remainder biscuit / After a voyage, he hath strange places crammed / With observation, the which he vents / In mangled forms" (II.vii.38–42). Both brains are made from a process of dislocation and displacement, from a voyaging that anatomizes the voyager. The result of "travels" is a brain crammed with bits and pieces that have lost their native ground, and with it, the anchor of their meaning. People become like those bits and pieces when they renounce their home to go wandering. Because all the exiles in Arden are wanderers, they are all vulnerable to such a loss of coherent identity. Apparently, the mechanism of "release" can undo the self by transforming it into "mangled forms," or a thing "compounded of many simples." This transformation ruins forms rather than renewing them.

Jaques and Touchstone, two characters Shakespeare added to his version of Lodge's "Rosalynde," use their unstructuring energies to expose the artificiality of the "nature" of Arden. Jaques, says Orlando, is a "fool or a cipher" and Touchstone is both. A cipher is a figure that increases or decreases the value of other figures though it is nothing in itself. It is everything and nothing like Jaques's melancholy. A touchstone is a catalyst of no value in itself which tests the value and authenticity of other things. Touchstone and Jaques, like Rosalind and Orlando, thus have a negative relation to the symbolic order—only in the formers' case they have a negative relation to the symbolic order of *Arden*. The nature of Arden, as well as the nature of society, is apparently inauthentic and unnatural. The good Duke Senior kills the natural inhabitants of the forest so that Jaques swears he does "more usurp" than his brother. And the duke further veils natural reality by translating it into a civilized style, by finding "tongues in trees, books in the running brooks / Sermons in stones, and good in everything" (II.i.16–17). His artificial means of representing nature does violence to nature— a "sweet style" usurps what it signifies.

The two "fools" point out the artificiality of the forest's inhabitants and devalorize the pastoral order so glorified by Duke Senior. William Empson has taught us what Jaques teaches in the forest ("most invectively he pierceth through the body of the country, city, court, yea, and of this our life, swearing that we are mere usurpers . . ."), that the pastoral world is an aristocratic invention tyrannically imposed on nature so that the court can claim the virtues of the simple life, the harmony between rich and poor, while keeping their distance from rustic life and smelly poverty.[11] Corin, the figure of this harsher nature, has hands that smell of tar not civet, and has known the cruelty of a churlish master. Jaques crows with delight when Touchstone cuts through the trappings of the pastoral ideal with his anato-

mizing wit and reveals an unidealized nature (itself a convention):

> . . . 'It is ten o'clock.
> Thus we may see,' quoth he, 'how the world wags.
> 'Tis but an hour ago since it was nine,
> And after one hour more 'twill be eleven;
> And so, from hour to hour, we ripe and ripe,
> And then, from hour to hour, we rot and rot;
> And therby hangs a tale.'
> (II.vii.22–28)

Touchstone reveals an ability to argue in "good set terms" juxtaposed with a belief that the world is sunk in meaningless matter.
This cynical view seems to be a product of the self-conscious
linguistic virtuosity that characterizes Touchstone and Jaques.
Their sophisticated attention to rhetoric has taught them that
words are dissociated from any absolute ground of meaning: the
matter of words mirrors the matter of the world which ripens
and rots. But though both Touchstone and Jaques expose the
unnatural nature of the symbolic order, Rosalind distinguishes
between them, and Touchstone is included in the comic order at
the end of the play while Jaques remains outside it.

When Rosalind says to Jaques, "I had rather have a fool to
make me merry than experience to make me sad," she indicates
that the fool accommodates man to society in a way that Jaques
does not. This seems odd at first because Touchstone is more
skeptical than Jaques. He is not nostalgic for a golden age and
claims no vision of moral perfection as the incentive for his
mocking attacks on the inhabitants of the court and forest. Paradoxically, Touchstone's skepticism is exactly what makes him
less disruptive than Jaques. Because he accepts all forms and
models of reality as equally true or false, he anatomizes the
world not to "cure" it but to provide entertaining proofs of the
illogic of logical analysis. Touchstone makes reason as strange
as madness, nature as absurd as courtly artifice. It is this unavoid-
able duplicity of our perceptions that redeems them. One cannot lie if one cannot speak the truth: ". . . if you swear by

that that is not, you are not forsworn" (I.ii.70–71). He cele-
brates the topsy-turvy condition of the world in which "the
truest poetry is the most feigning."[12] By radically separating the
fictional order from "true" reality he releases us from the burden
of trying to find the truth. Yet at the same time his "foolishness"
gives other characters a "seriousness," a measure of reality. In
this way, he prevents revelations about the artificial nature of
the comic order from turning the play into a tragic exploration
of the limits of symbolic order.

Touchstone finds the essential fictionality of the world a source
of freedom, Jaques finds it a source of melancholy. When Jaques
asks to be granted the role of fool, there is a proviso to his
request:

> It is my only suit,
> Provided that you weed your better judgments
> Of all opinion that grows rank in them
> That I am wise. I must have liberty
> Withal, as large a charter as the wind,
> To blow on whom I please. . . .
> (II.vii.44–49)

Jaques can only cleanse the "foul body of the infected world"
by distancing himself from all the false forms that give shape
to human experience; even the suit of the fool might constrain
him. This movement of separation challenges the value of the
refined comic order—and it undermines Jaques's own identity.
Liberty from an external identity means a self scattered to the
winds. By refusing any role, Jaques can have no stable identity;
by refusing any single system of interpretation, he can find the
world only in bits and pieces without relation or relevance. His
very name, Jaques, is associated with "jakes," a privy, and the
useless debris of man.

As far as Jaques is concerned, human forms are no more than
such debris. From his melancholy perspective, the body is a
locus of corruption, not of positive values. In his speech on the
seven ages of man, Jaques conducts a dissection of the body of
human life that gradually reduces it to nothing: "mere oblivion,
sans teeth, sans eyes, sans taste, sans everything" (II.vii.165–66).

Human reality is hollow, empty, because it is mere appearance: "All the world's a stage / And all the men and women merely players" (II.vii.139–40). Through the equation of the world and the stage, life and representation are conflated into superficial matter.[13] The coincidence of reality and the stage draws attention to the superficiality of Jaques's own language so his critique both loses some of its force and is strengthened by example: his melancholy posturing and verbal excesses, such as moralizing a spectacle into a "thousand similes," makes linguistic and theatrical representation seem unnatural and contrived. His anatomizing discourse is as limited and conventional as Orlando's love poetry—Orlando is "Signior Love," Jaques is another stereotype, "Monsieur Melancholy."[14] It is not "experience" or nature that has made Jaques sad, but books.[15] Orlando rebukes Jaques for his bookishness, saying, "I answer your right painted cloth, from whence you have studied your questions" (III.ii. 261–62). R. Warwick Bond insists that *Euphues* is the book that determines Jaques's identity: "Jaques . . . is simply Euphues Redivivus."[16] But Jaques also has much in common with Nashe—he negates forms (the bodies of country, city, court) to produce them. Jaques sucks life out of forms, as a "weasel sucks eggs" because the destruction of forms enables him to create new, fragmented ones.

If the decomposition of forms is a means of artistic production rather than a means of analysis, we might conclude that anatomy, or other means of "release," pose no real critique of the symbolic order. In a sense this is right, comedies mock the orders that serve for reality but also reinstate them as guarantors of community and proof of the existence of an irreducible meaning. But this comedy does not just pretend to desire "release" while actually firmly upholding the status quo. It is not enough to say that Jaques is merely a showman rather than a critic, and that Rosalind's effort to explore the depths is merely a ruse of language. Rosalind and Orlando insist that the social order of Duke Ferdinand is repressive; Jaques insists that man is encased in matter that separates him from the profound truth of things. And when the play ends, it is left to Jaques to expose the inadequacies of the "clarified" order of comic resolution. When he puts the characters in their places they begin to seem like

empirical objects: they are "you," "you," "you," "you," and "you."
By "you" he designates the Duke, Orlando, Oliver, Silvius, and
Touchstone, who are all lost to a form that usurps their identity.
The women are not designated at all. This comic form that
envelops the characters is no more absolute than the one created
by the usurping Duke Ferdinand; it will decay in time. Jaques
tells Touchstone: "Thy loving voyage is but for two months
victualled." What seems like a permanent order is yet another
voyage.

Jaques's refusal to succumb to any one vision of order, no
matter how compelling it is, seems misanthropic: he gives up
participation in a community in order to inhabit the duke's
abandoned cave. Yet the whole play has emphasized the affirmative power of negating forms and going into exile. A sign of
"true love" is a man's separation from society: "if thou hast not
broke from company / Abruptly . . . thou hast not loved" (II.
iv.37–39). Freedom is found in banishment, love in solitude,
life in Arden is "more sweet than that of painted pomp" (II.i.
2–3). As the lovers move back to court, new exiles inhabit the
forest, and this means what it did in the beginning—the need
for order is challenged by a desire to escape from its constraints.
Admittedly Duke Ferdinand is oddly cast as a "convertite" (yet
so is Oliver) and Jaques is a rather gloomy model of intellectual
liberty. But though each man's antidote for idolatry is extreme,
the play insists on the importance of subverting conventional
orders, even affirmative conventions of ending.

Though Jaques's refusal to join the dance of marriage may
seem to be a rejection of life, his renunciation gives expression
to the comedy's central desire for "release," a desire whose ability
to endanger comic order is now apparent. The tension we feel
between the comic celebration of form and the desire to escape
it is different from the *balance* between these two impulses that
is found in *Euphues* and "Euphues golden legacie." A mark of
this difference is its ability to produce tragedy. *As You Like It*
is a point of departure for a voyage into the fragmented world
of *King Lear*. Within the comic desire for a "clarified" order
grows a desperate need to reveal the essence of love and truth
that provokes and sustains the circular and disruptive anatomiz-

ing activity. Because an order "as you like it" is not the same as an order "as it really is" the play leaves us asking questions: Is man enslaved by false orders? Do these orders protect us from chaos? Can we anatomize these structures that bind us? Or should we?

5 · *Anatomy as Tragedy*

IN A DISCUSSION of *Julius Caesar,* Sigurd Burckhardt suggests that destruction is a tragic form of creation: "A tragedy—to define it very simply—is a *killing poem;* it is designed toward the end of bringing a man to some sort of destruction. And the killer is, quite literally, the poet; it is he, and no one else, who devises the deadly plot; it is he, therefore, who must in some sense accept responsibility for it."[1] In *King Lear* most of the killing is done by dismemberment; bodies are torn, wrenched, pierced, burst, broken, cracked, scourged, and flayed.[2] The physicality and destructiveness of acts of revelation in the play are captured in the term "anatomy," which describes both a technique of discovery and a torturous process of dismemberment. Bodies are anatomized in order to make their depths visible and comprehensible, but this process of externalization transforms the coherent "heart of things" into fragmented matter: by stripping away a body to reveal its contents the inside becomes the outside.

In abstract terms, this equivalence of inside and outside means that hidden values are exposed as fragmented matter and that fragmented matter becomes a source of truth. The effort to expose the moral condition of the world by anatomizing it thus ends by supporting an empiricist ideology whose truth seem to be mere surface. John Danby discusses the shift from a metaphysical to an empirical conception of "Nature" in a commentary on Lear's speech requesting an anatomy of Regan: "Then let them anatomize Regan. See what breeds about her heart. Is there any cause in nature that makes these hard hearts?" (III.vi.74–76). Danby comments that here the concept of "Nature" is "pushed across an important threshold. The physical nature of science (the Nature Bacon most concerns himself with in *Novum Organum*) is made to encroach upon the territory of moral corruption. For strict orthodoxy the Fall of man rather than anatomy should have been brought into the explanation." He goes on to connect the unexpected intrusion of anatomy into the realm of theology with the explorations of the world conducted by English entrepreneurs:

> Behind the shift and drift of the meanings of the word "Nature" there is the shift and drift of humanity in a setting at once historical and spiritual. . . . Behind Shakespeare there is the mining engineer breaking into the bowels of the earth; the seeker out of the mysteries of brass, and glass, and salt, and the supplier of the Elizabethan navies; the doctor taking apart the human body to anatomize the mechanism of muscle and bone; the capitalist aware of money as the . . . circulating life-blood of the body politic.[3]

Although this enthusiastic discussion is prompted by Lear's request for an anatomy, Danby ends up asserting that it illustrates the energy motivating Edmund's concept of "nature." By confusing the views of Lear and Edmund, Danby reveals his entanglement in the vertiginous movement of the play: past and future collide, the concepts of moral and empirical nature converge.

Rhetorically, the convergence of opposites generates paradoxes—and *Lear*, as everyone knows, is full of paradoxes. Less apparent is the affiliation between paradox and the method of anatomy. The paradox is a figure that disrupts the unity of discourse, of thought itself, by continually subverting the integrity of its own assertions about the world. Because it always ruptures itself, the contradictions that make up a paradox are not dialectical; they never resolve themselves in a synthesis. The process of anatomy is paradoxical because it both is and isn't a way of uncovering the truth. Although it is motivated by a faith that the mysterious essence of objects can be made visible, each moment of revelation also fragments the integrity of things. In a broad sense, *Lear* is about the paradoxes of this dismembering mode of representation: it demonstrates how a process of ordering can obliterate unity and a process of decomposition can compose a world.

Rosalie Colie, writing on seventeenth-century paradox, underscores the connection between the ambivalent, discontinuous structure of the play and paradox when she asserts that in *Lear* paradox is "normative." This statement implies that the norm has become one that transgresses norms, although Colie's interpretation of her own insight defuses the violence of the concept of paradox as a norm: she says that in *Lear* we see how paradox is used "to assert rather than to question moral and ethical standards."[4] How can this be so if paradox "plays back and forth across terminal boundaries"?[5] Her attempt to moralize paradox imitates the efforts of the play's characters to control the continuous shifting of one thing into its opposite ("nothing," for example, into "all") by contriving an exemplum or, in this case, an exemplary figure, which will control the meaning of the action.[6] But the effort to impose a moral interpretation has an effect opposed to the one intended; the imposition of order contributes to disorder. Trying to maintain order, Lear fragments his kingdom; Gloucester's attempt to interpret Edgar leads him to violate his son's integrity and his own; Cordelia and Edgar humiliate their fathers in order to restore their dignity. Paradox is indeed the norm in this play, and this means that ethical standards are undermined by asserting them.

This merger of opposites which defies a positive meaning is also a fragmentation: the self that becomes not itself loses its integrity. The two masters of paradox in the play, Lear and the Fool, suffer the radical disintegration of self that results when identity is equated with nonidentity: both of them are things of nothing. After completing Lear's paradoxical "We'll go to supper i'th'morning" with "And I'll go to bed at noon," the Fool goes off the stage and never comes back, and Lear dissolves into a madness that is the only possible "knowledge" of the paradoxical state of his world:

A man may see how this world goes with no eyes. Look
with thine ears. See how yond justice rails upon yond
simple thief. Hark in thine ear: change places and, handy-
dandy, which is the justice, which is the thief? (IV.vi.
148–52)

In this topsy-turvy world where ears replace eyes, opposites such
as a justice and a thief change places and yet retain their own
identity; a sense of division remains even though the lines between criminality and justice are blurred. The fragmentation of
order does not lead to a total rupturing of barriers that would
return men to a primal unity, to a paradisaical wholeness. The
pathos of the world of paradox is caused by this inability to
effect true union through fragmentation; its horror lies in the
threat that such a union might take place and destroy the values
maintained through the opposition of good and evil, truth and
falsehood, order and disorder.

The pathos of the method of anatomy is never more apparent
than when it makes human identity precarious by confusing self
and nonself. In terms of personal identity, the equation of inside and outside that results from anatomizing a subject means
that the interior of the self is dispersed into a fragmented external form in order to be revealed. The anatomy of a body is
thus an act of destruction and of revelation. And often the
anatomy that reveals something of an external body acts to destroy the anatomist. For example, Cordelia exposes the inadequacy of Lear's regal discourse, a discourse masquerading as
truth which allows Lear to pose as the master of all reality. He
responds by calling her a "little seeming substance." But this
reduction of her is a sign of his own disintegration; Kent inter-
prets it as proof that "Lear is mad." In this way the breaking up
of Lear's identity is linked to his efforts to obliterate Cordelia.
What is outside, and seemingly other, is also a mirror of the
self. Because they cruelly reduce their childlike father from king
to "poor forked animal," Regan and Goneril are demonic images
of Lear as well as the source of his destruction. They also express
the negative side of Cordelia's critique of her father. This dis-
sociation of bad attributes of good characters gives the play its

allegorical dimension.[7] Regan and Goneril personify evil forces of destruction; the positive side of the process of disintegration, the side represented by Cordelia, is its ability to bring about self-knowledge. As Lear strips away his own pomp and pretensions, he approaches the truths that Cordelia insists exist beyond the masks of language and public ritual. He can only approach them, however, for the anatomizing process impedes its own ends by obliterating what it reveals.

It is in the nature of tragic drama that the poet cannot achieve a final dramatization of positive absolute truth because he insists that the world of appearances, of the theater, be fragmented. One way Shakespeare accomplishes the fragmentation of dramatic form is by deleting the motives for the action that were provided in the earlier drama of *King Lear*. For this reason Tolstoy preferred the older play and Nahum Tate rewrote Shakespeare's version to provide it with an order acceptable to a bourgeois audience as Shakespeare's tragic, disruptive form was not.[8] Lear is an anatomy, a kind of antiform; Tate constructed a happily positive form. A. C. Bradley is sympathetic with Tate's effort because he believes the play is not a dramatic whole. According to him, the mass of material it includes, the vagueness of its temporality and location, the lack of causal order (the ending, for example, seems unjustified), all make the play "imperfectly dramatic."[9] This judgment follows traditional theory, based on a dubious reading of Aristotle's *Poetics,* which states that a dramatist should use time and place to unify a play and allow it to imitate nature.[10] But Shakespeare uses the "unities" of time and space as instruments of fragmentation, as the means to get beyond artificial forms to nature. The time of anatomy is the time of decay; decay dissolves the ground of the action.

The temporal movement of the play has a double and antagonistic function: it both unfolds the truth and undermines it. Cordelia, for example, tells her sisters that "time shall unfold what plighted cunning hides," but the temporal process of exposure is as much involved in the destruction of a moral order as in its restoration. Yet, although the villains of the play take advantage of the time to kill Cordelia, time does not allow them to maintain a position of mastery. They too are destroyed in time, but not because time is redemptive. The temporal process of the drama interferes with efforts to structure it, to interpret it as either progressive or destructive, by what Elton calls "sequential ironies." Each effort to impose a causal or moral order on the action of the play is undercut, exposed in time, "like a series of trapdoors."[11] Edgar moralizes hopefully, "The worst returns to laughter" (IV.i.6), and the blinded Gloucester wanders on stage; Albany's prayer, "The gods defend her" (V.iii.258) is answered by the presentation of Cordelia's dead body. But these examples are almost too familiar, they domesticate the disruptive power of time. The maddeningly antithetical nature of time in the play is perhaps best enunciated by the Fool. He describes an ambivalent utopia, a nowhere in which the good become bad and the bad become good, and then locates himself as speaker in an inconceivable time: "This prophecy Merlin shall make, for I live before his time" (III.ii.95–96). Here future and past are confused, as are negative and positive views of history. Time, in its linear aspect, is not a category that can be used to structure a conclusive unifying meaning for the play.

The disruptive process of time is intensified by a loss of coherence in space. The characters are literally homeless; they have lost their place because the customary hierarchical order is shattered. The houseless Lear accompanied by the Fool is never in the same place twice; Gloucester wanders vaguely toward Dover, arriving only at a Dover that does not really exist; Regan and Cornwall leave home to avoid Lear, Goneril to find him; and even more peripatetic than all the others are Edgar and Kent. These moving particles present an image of an atomized world in which all are detached from an original ground. The movements of the characters are arbitrary, no longer governed by a moral teleology. Hence the questions that critics keep asking about the peregrinations of the characters are inevitable—but unanswerable: What happened to France? Why does Gloucester go to Dover and why does he send Lear there? Where does the Fool go? What business is Kent upon that makes it necessary for him to refuse Cordelia's request that he take off his disguise? Critics wish to place characters in a text that displaces the very idea of place. The incessant wanderings of the characters, the use of a nonplace like the heath as the center of the action, work to undermine the idea of space as a dramatic "unity."

The characters are not so much headed for a particular goal as they are in flight from real or imagined persecutors and from their own acts of violence. In the name of "love," "nature," or "reason," all the inhabitants of the world of *King Lear* commit acts of aggression toward others, acts designed to reduce their victims to nothing. Even an incomplete litany of such offenses is a long one: Cordelia and Kent attack Lear's public role; Lear banishes Cordelia and strips her of her property and his benediction; Gloucester violently proceeds against Edgar; Edmund betrays his father; Cornwall stamps out Gloucester's eyes and Edgar keeps him in darkness; Albany threatens to dismember his wife; Goneril and Regan strip away the king's retainers; Lear inflicts them with blasting curses. This catalog of destruction reveals that each act of violence returns to harm the aggressor. (Edgar, Kent, and Albany survive to the end of the play only at the cost of what they value.) This is not so much a mechanism of justice but of total annihilation: "Humanity must perforce prey on itself, / Like monsters of the deep" (IV.ii.48–49).

This mechanism, like the method of anatomy, makes the process of revelation a process of destruction. The characters, then, as well as the dramatist, are anatomists: they strip away masks, penetrate and fragment the body. We must turn to the play to learn the particular ways in which an anatomy disrupts and displaces the solidity of things. How does it disrupt the body politic? What is its effect on language? On knowledge itself?

The play begins with a ritualized act of division meant to insure the survival of the body politic, or as Lear puts it, to prevent "further strife." I regard Lear's kingdom as a "body politic" because it is the fundamental concept of political order prior to the eighteenth century. The idea of the body politic presupposes an organic coherence among all the members of a state. This political body is a mirror of the divine body of Christ, linked to the body politic through the sovereign who heads both church and state. Lear's decision to give each of his children an equal share of the kingdom violates the law of primogeniture and the principles of monarchy and hierarchy that are the ancient sources of legitimacy for the body politic. The obliteration of these principles simultaneously disintegrates the metaphysical values associated with the body politic and the body of the king through the traditional correspondence between the secular and divine orders. Lear does this unconscious violence to his world because he uses the fragmenting methods of an anatomist to order it. Not only does his technique of ordering cause the disintegration of his kingdom, it also precipitates the breakdown of his family. The love test can be seen as an anatomizing device that will allow Lear to see what his family is really made of, to expose the real natures of his daughters. But rather than putting things into order by dividing them into parts and penetrating to their depths, Lear dissolves his kingdom and his family, and exposes the disruptive power of the anatomizing process.

The immediate consequence of Lear's reductive strategy of ordering is the separation of social forms from customary values. In the process of uncovering the essential nature of his society, Lear externalizes it, turns it into fragmented visible matter. This matter has no relation to the unified mystic corpus that consecrates the body politic and the body royal. The king, as Kantorowicz puts it, is left a "physis now devoid of any metaphysis" and language too is hollowed out because words are detached from the original ground of their meaning.[12] The language of love and loyalty that Goneril and Regan speak is cut off from the virtues of love and loyalty. As a result of Lear's action these virtues have become unspeakable—separate and silent, they are like Cordelia.

Cordelia cannot speak positive values so she says "nothing" and points to the limits of courtly rhetoric: "I want that glib and oily art / To speak and purpose not" (I.i.224-25). She articulates the separation between speech and its referent to persuade her father to penetrate beyond words to get at the formless essences of love and loyalty he asks for. Language must be stripped away to be redeemed, an anatomizing approach to redemption that intensifies the process of fragmentation already begun by Lear. Cordelia, Lear says later, "wrenched my frame of nature / From the fixed place" (I.iv.259-60). Kent, by calling himself Lear's "physician," also attempts to bring Lear to himself by stripping away his public role: "What wouldst thou do, old man?" (I.i.146). Cordelia's plainness and Kent's rudeness are methods to cut away the superfluities that stand between Lear and the truth and thus return Lear and his kingdom to their proper order. But that customary order is gone, so the process of stripping away masks promises to reduce Lear to nothing, a cipher, a dead man. In other words, although Cordelia and Kent anatomize Lear as an act of love, in doing so they repeat Lear's disruptive act of ordering. Even those with the "best meaning" have "incurred the worst" (V.iii.4).

The disturbing similarity between the methods of discovery used by Lear and Cordelia reveals the struggle in the play about whether or not the method of anatomy should be conceived as negative or positive. On the one hand, the anatomist's way to get at truth has the negative effect of separating appearances from truth. Cordelia, because she says nothing and is given nothing, represents that estranged truth: "Truth," Lear says, is her "dower" (I.i.108). France and Kent attach themselves to the truth by defending Cordelia; apparently Lear must find truth by negating the devalued forms and masks that keep it hidden. Yet the process of stripping away forms has already been shown to lead not *to* the truth but *away* from it—Lear's effort to get at the center of things has disrupted the ground of his world. To reach the unifying center Cordelia represents, he must destroy her. The refusal to attempt a reconciliation, however, has equally bad effects; it leaves him stranded in a fragmented world, controlled by Goneril and Regan, where he will be destroyed.

The Fool describes how Cordelia's absence causes fragmentation: "after I have cut the egg i'th' middle and eat up the meat" two empty shells remain. We are left with the "parings." Gloucester paints a picture of this exploded world: "Love cools, friendship falls off, brothers divide. In cities, mutinies; in countries, discord; in palaces, treason; and the bond cracked 'twixt son and father" (I.ii.104–8). Only the universality of contradiction unites the warring parties: kings and subjects, fathers and sons, young and old. As Lyly's insistently antithetical anatomy demonstrates, a world locked in violent opposition is both created and discovered by the process of anatomizing. In Lyly's work antithesis makes absolute the separation between one object and another; but in *Lear,* paradox subverts opposites by placing extremes together so that they transgress each other, rupturing the wholeness of opposed bodies, and leveling differences. Roland Barthes, in a discussion of these figures, explains how paradox can be used to cross the bar between antithesis:

> The several hundred figures propounded by the art of rhetoric down through the centuries constitute a labor of classification intended to name, to lay the foundations for, the world. Among all these figures, one of the most stable is the Antithesis; its apparent function is to consecrate (and domesticate) by a name, by a metalinguistic object, the division between opposites and the very irreducibility of this division. The antithesis separates for eternity; it thus refers to a nature of opposites, and this nature is untamed. Far from differing merely by the presense or lack of a simple relationship (as is ordinarily the case with paradigmatic opposites), the two terms of an antithesis are each *marked:* their difference does not arise out of a complementary, dialectical movement (empty as opposed to full): the antithesis is the figure of the *given* opposition, eternal, eternally recurrent: the figure of the inexpiable. Every joining of two antithetical terms, every mixture, every conciliation—in short, every passage through the wall of Antithesis—constitutes a transgression; to be sure, rhetoric can reinvent a figure designed to name the transgressive; this figure exists; it is the *paradoxism* (or alliance of words): an unusual figure, it is the code's ultimate attempt to affect the inexpiable.[13]

In *Lear,* opposites transgress each other through the paradox of anatomy that links order and disorder, forces of good and forces of evil.

In the first act, for example, Goneril and Regan clearly demonstrate the violence and disruption associated with the methods of ordering already employed by Lear and Cordelia. They act "i'th'heat," exercising a passionate energy much like Lear's, to undo Lear's power so it cannot strip away their authority and position. In using techniques of anatomizing to consolidate their state, they mirror Lear, and through this mirroring, show us the complicity between good and evil in the play. The "bad" sisters, like Lear, Cordelia, and Kent, present their anatomy as a social good; Goneril and Regan will strip away Lear's retainers who "Do hourly carp and quarrel" in order to protect the body politic, the "wholesome weal" (I.iv.201) and their own authority which Lear threatens to divide "under two commands."[14] They claim that their own bodies are also endangered by Lear and his knights. Goneril tells her husband that Lear "may enguard his dotage" with the power of his knights and "hold our lives in mercy" (I.iv.317–18); Regan repeats her sister's fears when she announces that Lear "is attended with a desperate train, / And what they may incense him to, being apt / To have his ear abused, wisdom bids fear" (II.iv.300–302). In cutting their father's train, scanting his sizes, and shutting the bolt against his coming in, they ostensibly act to create order. Like Lear dividing his kingdom, they act to insure the safety of the realm. If we don't accept this explanation, it is because we can see now how self-serving the violent imposition of order can be. As Foucault has labored to show, the sovereign power to impose order violently exerts itself on the bodies of those it orders—it anatomizes them. This violent spectacle of order can be interpreted as a triumph of truth, or as an act of atrocity.[15]

Goneril and Regan mask the disruptive power of ordering by insisting that the cause of disorder lies outside themselves, beyond even Lear's control, because the source of corruption is his body, an external form subject to the "infirmities of his age." By proposing a physical cause, old age, as the basis of Lear's behavior, Regan and Goneril translate Lear's desires into the irrational products of his body's decay. This dehumanizing reduction of human desires to a physiological function is both a consequence of, and a justification for, anatomizing a body. The materialist claim that all knowledge can be made visible justifies a search for discrete facts. Anatomizing is a method of appropriating the truth, of making facts visible, by tearing a total body into pieces. These pieces, created and discovered by the anatomist, confirm the beliefs that motivate scientific anatomies in the first place. The propensity to reduce men and nature to measurable, quantifiable, visible phenomena is anticipated by Lear who maps his kingdom and tries to quantify love, and is fully embodied by his daughters. Goneril and Regan make Lear conform to his "objective" condition by stripping away the superfluities that disguise his age and decrepitude. The empiricist conception of reality that informs their acts also determines the language that they speak, the language of "facts."[16] The violence associated with the assumption of a style as objective as nature itself points out the destructiveness of the reduction of man and nature on which the ideology of objectivity is based. In the interests of "reason" Goneril and Regan commit acts of violence that appear unnatural and mad, just as Lear, to protect his sovereign word, must foolishly attack Cordelia and Kent. "How far your eyes may pierce I cannot tell," Albany remarks to Goneril, "Striving to better, oft we mar what's well' (I.v.336–37).

In this play acts of seeing, of representing reality, lead to blindness and confusion.[17] This accounts for the many paradoxical images of sight. Lear and Gloucester, as well as Goneril and Regan, desire to spatialize all knowledge, to make things clear and visible. Gloucester, who believes in "evidence" that will insure his ability to interpret reality correctly, and Lear, who denies the existence of the invisible truths Cordelia points to, share Goneril and Regan's blind faith in "facts." Faith in the power literally to see the truth is a sign of blindness of the inner eye, insight. Lear's daughters never "see" the inadequacy of the order of truth they violently impose on reality; Lear and Gloucester "see" limits in their former ways of seeing only when they no longer have the power to prescribe the conditions of order that are to be taken as nature itself. On the heath, cut off from the grounding power of his former authority, Lear recognizes the tyranny of order, for now it is his identity that is denied by those in power in order to maintain the status quo. His insight into the conditions of order is paradoxically a product of his madness. The limits of reason and facts are understood by the madman because his madness places him beyond the boundaries of logic and order. In "eyeless rage," in the absence of reason, Lear sees how the world goes. Gloucester's blindness brings him literally closer to the world, for he sees it "feelingly," a bit at a time. Things are clarified as fictions of totality slip away. The blindness and cruelty of the eye that anatomizes the world in the effort to make it subservient to reason is replaced with the vision of darkness and madness that returns man to the incomprehensible fullness of nature.

Goneril and Regan cannot reach this extreme and yet central place where reason and unreason mingle. The illusion of their autonomy from the objects exposed to their piercing eyes keeps them separate. Yet if this illusion stops self-reflection and a confrontation with the inadequacy of their mode of knowing, it does not protect them from the consequence of their disruptive way of seeing things. As Albany tells Goneril, her attack on her father's integrity is simultaneously an act of self-mutilation, of uprooting. His description of this process suggests that the destruction of an origin, a father, anatomizes its issue:

> That nature which condemns its origin
> Cannot be bordered certain in itself.
> She that herself will sliver and disbranch
> From her material sap, perforce must wither
> And come to deadly use.
> (IV.ii.32–36)

By cutting down their father, Goneril and Regan initiate their own disintegration, which has no value as a means of redemption. Lear, the object of their anatomy, presents a more optimistic picture of the method of anatomy because his fragmentation is connected with a movement toward self-knowledge.

Lear feels the reduction of his knights from one hundred to none as a process of physical disintegration. Goneril's talk of it pierces his heart, her tongue strikes him and strips him of his "manhood." Her words evidently have the power of acts of murder and castration (he bursts into womanly sobs) which cause a humiliating loss of self. His answer to these cutting words is a promise of revenge and a self-pitying assertion that he did nothing to provoke the assault on his body. This claim of innocence helps validate the release of formless violence that breaks through his language:

> I will have such revenges on you both
> That all the world shall—I will do such things—
> What they are, yet I know not; but they shall be
> The terrors of the earth.
> (II.iv.274–77)

Lear exalts the negative animus behind his attack on Regan and Goneril as a moral force that is authorized by nature. He prefaces his curse of Goneril by saying, "Hear, Nature, hear; dear Goddess, hear"—words disturbingly reminiscent of Edmund's "Thou, Nature, art my goddess; to thy law / My services are bound." Kent also insists that violence can be justified in a good cause because in such cases, "Anger hath a privilege." But this conventional argument for the use of violence can be turned around. Cornwall reiterates the freedoms allowed to anger before he blinds Gloucester: "our power / Shall do a court'sy to our wrath which men / May blame, but not control" (III.vii.24–26). By violently dismembering violent enemies ("no contraries," remarks Kent about Oswald, "hold more antipathy than I and such a knave") one expands the domain of violence and fragmentation. Even violence in the interest of good doubles back on itself. As Laurence Michel points out, Cornwall "does not merely blast Kent with unthinking retaliatory fury, but anatomizes the defects of his virtue in its genuine aspects as well":

> These kind of knaves I know, which in this plainness
> Harbor more craft and more corrupter ends
> Than twenty silly-ducking observants
> That stretch their duties nicely.
> (II.ii.96–99)[18]

Kent's violent anatomy of Oswald is a sign of his own corruption, and lands him in the stocks; Cornwall's fury leads to his violent death, the "chance of anger." In the case of Cornwall, the way that an anatomy savagely folds back to cut the anatomist seems a mechanism of poetic justice. But this mechanism also turns the supposedly just acts of Kent into criminal ones that must be punished. The inversion of the process of anatomy thus confuses the higher and lower aims of the anatomist. Even Lear's dissection of his evil daughters leads to his own exhaustion and disintegration.

Lear uses words as instruments to dismember his daughters. The curse or tongue-lashing is an ancient form of mutilation, which Mary Claire Randolph connects to the use of medical imagery by Renaissance critics and satirists who anatomize, cut, burn, and blister the bodies of their subjects, ostensibly to cure them of their sins.[19] Lear's vocabulary of dismemberment has no such therapeutic intent; he wants to "kill, kill, kill, kill, kill, kill." Without a goal, his desire for destruction is destined to be as repeatedly manifested as the word "kill" and to become an end in itself. At the close of the play, Lear is still obsessively trying to affect destruction: "Had I your tongues and eyes, I'ld use them so / That heaven's vault should crack" (V.iii.259–60). As we have seen, both "good" and "bad" characters sanction such cosmic destruction by making it "natural"—nature performs the anatomizing of tongues and eyes. Lear calls upon nature to make Goneril sterile, and to give his words the power to "pierce every sense about her." Regan, he promises, will flay her "wolvish visage" with her nails. And it is nature's voice, thunder, that should anatomize the whole world, "crack Nature's mold" and "rive concealing continents." In this way nature becomes an anatomizing discourse that disrupts the order of nature itself.

The simultaneous presence of nature as the image of human and divine order and as the source of its destruction provides a bridge between Lear's traditional curses of Goneril and his modernist request for an anatomy of Regan. An anatomy will accomplish a fragmentation of Regan's body comparable to the fragmentation of her sister's body that Lear wants to accomplish with his curses. But by using an anatomy instead of a curse, Lear adopts the rationale for violence employed by his daughters to justify their attack on his body: the anatomy of a body is equated with the search for objective truth. If Lear can discover an empirical "cause" for human action or "hard hearts," then he can displace the origin of human violence from man, from the anatomist, to nature itself.[20] Such a displacement subverts the traditional idea of nature as a benign and virtuous order, yet by excluding disorder from the human domain men hope to isolate and master the essential violence of nature and of themselves. Shakespeare, who conspicuously assigns an empiricist mode of seeing and speaking to the villains of the play, apparently does not believe that empiricist modes of knowing will lead to the creation of an order more absolute and grounded than the old order of microcosm and macrocosm whose place it usurps. Goneril, Regan, and Edmund obstruct the establishment of a unified truth because their mode of ordering is based on the fragmentation rather than the integration of nature and culture. The empiricist ideology, however, does offer a positive interpretation of a fragmented universe which otherwise appears to be an incomprehensible sphere of chaos and madness. Lear's request for an anatomy to discover the cause of hard hearts is thus a last attempt to preserve himself from that flux, but an attempt that, like his efforts to unify his kingdom by dividing it, only abets the forces of decay.

The etymology of the word "decay" links the domains of the spirit and the body. Its root is a Latin compound of *de* (down) plus *cadere* (to fall) which means "to fall." A falling, a rupturing of unity constitutes the temporality of the drama and describes the tragedy of Lear himself. Albany calls him "this great decay" (V.iii.298). In effect, decay is the essence of the order of this play; it is as inhumanly fertile as a rotting corpse that "smells of mortality." The fragmentation of an organic whole creates a degraded life whose power is linked with animality and sexuality. Lear compares Regan and Goneril to animals that rip into the body (darting serpents, gnawing rats, biting dogs) and to beasts that feed on the decay of bodies ("sharp-toothed" vultures, "detested" kites). This animal aggression is identified with sexuality which Lear describes as a destructive not a creative force. In his harangue against sexuality as an anatomizing energy, Lear strips away the clothes that cover a woman's body to reveal a form that is not as virginal as "snow" but a source of corruption: "hell," "darkness," "stench," and "consumption" are located "down from the waist" (IV.vi.118–28). His preceding remarks to Gloucester show that he realizes how such a passionate anatomy of women reveals the erotic desires of the anatomist who participates in the disintegrative energy of sexuality:

Thou rascal beadle, hold thy bloody hand!
Why dost thou lash that whore? Strip thy own back.
Thou hotly lusts to use her in that kind
For which thou whip'st her.
(IV.vi.157–60)

Opposites again converge; the whipping of a whore reveals the corrupt desires of the whipper. Lear's disgust at the beadle and his victim leaves him with no way out of the degraded sphere of the body because both erotic union and the refusal of it are signs of corrupt sexuality. Regan and Goneril feed off the decay of their father, Lear acquires energy from dismembering them. Decomposition is an inhuman form of creation.

The destructive form of creation is apparently nature's own. It is intolerable to watch Regan and Cornwall perform the vivisection of Gloucester which is also enacted in the play's language—he is plucked by the beard, hairs are ravished from his chin, his eyes are stamped out. But, although Gloucester's tortures seem unnaturally cruel, they mirror the action of nature on the heath. The "pelting" storm invades men to the skin and shatters the "little world of man." Time, space, and nature are as indifferent as Regan and Cornwall to the suffering they cause in the human sphere. All possess a metonymic power that flays the skin, cuts to the brains, and shatters reason and language. Yet the unintelligible parts created by this process have an elusive power because they make up the chaos from which all coherent forms are made. The contradictory equation of fragmentation and fertility not only imbues Edmund, Regan, and Goneril with sexual and animal energy, but it also fills madness with life: "Sa! Sa! Sa! Sa!" Lear's madness makes him a "natural." But this nature, as a source of fragmentation, is an obstacle that stands between Lear and the unifying values of love and bond. To reach Cordelia, he must go beyond nature to the verge of its confine: "You are a spirit, I know. Where did you die?" (IV.vii.49).

At the beginning of the play, Cordelia points out the necessity of going beyond public forms to grasp the spirit of love and bond. By putting off his "lendings" and taking off the false coverings of clothes, reason, and language, Lear comes close to the sublime truths Cordelia represents. But to attain this metaphysical "all" Lear has had to disperse himself into the world. The fullness of "all" descends to the emptiness of "nothing." He can no longer exist by anatomizing others—this destructive mode of life has exhausted his strength—so, at the verge of destruction, he can finally accept Cordelia's love. The connection between reunion and the loss of power is reinforced by the structure of the play: the scene of reconciliation between Cordelia and Lear is quickly followed by their appearance on the stage as prisoners. And the deadly conjunction of the extremes of joy and grief is enacted again in the death of Gloucester as Edgar describes it:

> his flaw'd heart—
> Alack, too weak the conflict to support—
> 'Twixt two extremes of passion, joy and grief,
> Burst smilingly.
> (V.iii.197–200)

Lear hopes the prison walls will form a body invulnerable to bursting. As "God's spies," he and Cordelia could then seek out daughters and sisters and pry into the secrets of the court without undergoing the disintegration of self that is linked in the world of this play to both the destructive and the therapeutic exposure of others. But there is no escaping the laws of this anatomizing universe; the outside becomes the inside, the inside the outside. Lear projects death on the decaying, fertile world outside the prison; but his prison "cage" is itself an inside place of death and decay. Cordelia is annihilated; the "thick rotundity of the world" is flattened as the center is again emptied out. Cordelia, "dead as earth," is totally objectified. The capture of the ideal leads back to the meaningless materiality of the world. To make values visible and present causes their disintegration. Their absence causes the disintegrating strife of all the bodies of society.

Cordelia's silent love, like the "unpublished virtues of the earth," maintains a coherent value by virtue of its separation from a fragmented and superficial public order. Since the anatomizing process fragments the interior of things to make them visible, it seems safer to keep the depths hidden. Edgar and Kent remain intact to the end of the play because they adopt disguises that keep their supposedly real and noble natures undisclosed and protected. Both men have pragmatic reasons for taking on a fictitious identity and maintaining it. Kent has been banished by the king whose acknowledgment he lives for—if he is seen, "that moment" is his death. Edgar has been sentenced to death by his father, so he is understandably reluctant to give him "eyes again" by revealing himself. The problem with disguises is that they compromise the virtues they are meant to protect—the loyal servant acts deviously and the good son contributes to his father's blindness—although without playing parts the two men could not survive. Lear confirms the utility of disguise as a means of preventing self-annihilation:

> Our basest beggars
> Are in the poorest thing superfluous.
> Allow not nature more than nature needs,
> Man's life is cheap as beast's.
> (II.iv.259–62)

To deny a man superfluities is to deny him human identity. Yet paradoxically, the disguises that protect identity also violate it: Edgar and Kent must alienate themselves from themselves by taking on a false identity. And because their "real" selves are always absent, neither seems to have a fixed essential self. In reality, they are all appearance. The closer Edgar and Kent get to nature, the more artificial they become—the rustic garb of Caius is Kent's disguise, Edgar disguises himself with nakedness.

Such a separation of role from self is exactly what initiates the tragedy in the first place. And it also initiates the desire to get at the truths that exist beyond superficial forms—that is, to anatomize. Edmund is the most evil character because he continually manipulates appearances by creating theater pieces. His dramas, the pat rivalry of Gloucester and Edgar, of Goneril and Regan, and his strategies of self (he slides from one pose to another) are effective theater inasmuch as they make a reality of appearances. The success of such simulacra puts into question the authenticity of all representations of reality, traditional forms as well as iconoclastic ones, and has radical consequences for the artist himself. As a result of stage-managing by both Lear and Edmund, the customary order is usurped and the world of the play is detached from any authentic ground. This negative view of theatricality contaminates everyone on the stage, even Cordelia. Cordelia's plainness and Lear's madness seem natural and honest in comparison to the contrived madness of Edgar and the stylized plainness of Kent. But the comparison that legitimizes Lear and Cordelia also has the negative effect of demonstrating the fictitiousness and conventionality of madness and honesty as they are presented in the theater. Like all forms of representation, drama fragments and reduces the most extreme and absolute of human experiences in order to represent them. We could say that all representation requires a limiting of what is limitless. In *King Lear,* Shakespeare attempts to open up the constraining limits of dramatic form so that he can reveal the plenitudes of nature and truth. But what he discovers is that by stripping away empty masks in an effort finally to present solid and coherent truths, he participates in a fragmenting process of representation while trying to circumvent it. The effort to get beyond the reductive properties of dramatic form by anatomizing them only enlarges the domain of fragmentation.

By attempting to go beyond the dramatic order, Shakespeare, like Lear, further collapses metaphysical values into fragmented empirical matter. His anatomizing mode of drama, which opens up the depths to our eyes and brings us close to the animal passions and the ideals of love and bond that exist beyond form, also requires the brutal disintegration of the bodies of man, the state, and his own media, language and drama. Both Cordelia's broken body and the king's own racked one show the cost of the desire to possess her and the truths she represents, even though Lear's mad dream that she still lives continues to promise that the formless essences of her breath, voice, and love can be externalized without destroying them. Shakespeare begins to write such dreams: Cleopatra's death is an erotic reunion, and in the late romances death dissolves into a fiction that conceals life. But on the stage of *Lear* the men who survive—Albany, Edgar, Kent—exist in roles deprived of substance.

That Cordelia's spirit has disintegrated into fragmented matter in order to make it visible affirms the Baconian dream that the only truths capable of surviving scrutiny are the dehumanized truths of material facts. This dream is given potency because of the way that the search for metaphysical truths inevitably leads back to fragmented matter. But the play exposes such matter as theatrical and an obstacle to truth. In *King Lear* Shakespeare makes the external world into a problem; it is a fictional body that must be anatomized to get at essential values, but which cannot be anatomized without destroying those values. With the help of an anatomizing method, Bacon tries to make the external world into an answer. The domain of drama slides into the domain of science; the world becomes an anatomical theater, the theater for the play of a medical science.

6 · Anatomy as Science

IT IS COMMONLY held that the publication of Sir Francis Bacon's *The Proficience and Advancement of Learning* in 1605 marks the end of the Renaissance and the beginning of our modern scientific era. Bacon would undoubtedly be pleased with this appraisal of his work, for he too believed that he was the inaugurator of a new era. His confidence in the novelty and value of his enterprise, the construction of a "true model of the world," is everywhere apparent, but never more so than when he talks to his fictional audience, the "sons of science." With the "sons" he does not mince his words: "I suppose that I have established forever a true and lawful marriage between the empirical and the rational faculty, the unkind and ill-starred divorce and separation of which has thrown into confusion the affairs of the human family" ("Preface" to *The Great Instauration,* 1:246).[1] Bacon's claims for himself are claims for his anatomizing method.

For Bacon, the metaphor of anatomy, not the more familiar one of the telescope, establishes a new "natural" relationship between man, language, and nature. His assured placement of an anatomical method and language within the order of truth and nature gave authority to the discipline of science and to himself as a founding father: "no man quite escapes his presence in the haunted building of science, or the whispers of his approbation or unease."[2] This voice still murmuring in the byways of science persistently adopts fragmenting modes of articulation—induction, antithesis, aphorisms, scientific tables—that apparently have the power to open up the world to the eyes of man. But by scrutinizing Bacon's discourse, we shall see that this alleged mastery of nature by science is yet another "idol" or "false apparition." Bacon's science remains wedded to language, as he was very much aware, and wedded to troublesome effects of anatomy that he cannot acknowledge because he believes he has language under complete control.

Earlier anatomists, as we have seen, ostensibly dissected the corrupt body of the world so that men could see the errors of their ways and reform their lives. Even Nashe, the most lawless of anatomists, conducts an anatomy of absurdity "that each one at first sight may eschew it as infectious, to shew it to the worlde that men may shunne it."[3] Bacon is said to be a harbinger of modernity because he puts the empirical technique of anatomizing to the work of investigating the material rather than the moral condition of the world. This change in the intention of the anatomist seems at first to be the result of a new view of the proper ends of knowledge. Bacon insists that the goal of his method is the discovery of the material components of nature, not its final cause, but he also claims that the discovery of the "Forms of things" is the key to interpreting the Book of Nature and hence he grounds his method in the old theological idea of nature as a book in which one can read the ultimate purpose of things.[4]

The complexity of Bacon's effort to establish the teleology of science is visible in a passage from the *Novum Organum* in which he announces his intention to conduct an "anatomy of the world." Its logic is compressed and apparently contradictory assertions are placed together as if there were no discontinuity between them. This stylistic feature makes the passage difficult to read but enables Bacon to attach his scientific project to a theological tradition, and, almost simultaneously, to attack that tradition. In this double movement the discourse of science acquires a metaphysical foundation and displaces traditional "philosophic systems" that formerly articulated the pathway toward truth. Here is the passage that concerns us:

Again, it will be thought, no doubt, that the goal and mark of knowledge which I myself set up (the very point at which I object to in others) is not the true or the best; for that the contemplation of truth is a thing worthier and loftier than all utility and magnitude of works; and that this long and anxious dwelling with experience and matter and the fluctuations of individual things, drags down the mind to earth or rather sinks it to a very Tartarus of turmoil and confusion; removing and withdrawing it from the serene tranquility of abstract wisdom, a condition far more heavenly. Now to this I readily assent; and indeed this which they point at as so much to be preferred, is the very thing of all other which I am about. For I am building in the human understanding a true model of the world, such as it is in fact, not such as man's own reason would have it to be; a thing which cannot be done without a very diligent dissection and anatomy of the world. But I say that those foolish and apish images of worlds which the fancies of men have created in philosophical systems, must be utterly scattered to the winds. Be it known how vast a difference there is (as I said above) between the Idols of the human mind and the Ideas of the divine. The former are nothing more than arbitrary abstractions; the latter are the Creator's own stamp upon creation, impressed and defined in matter by true and exquisite lines. Truth therefore and utility are here the very same things; and works themselves are of greater value as pledges of truth than as contributing to the comforts of life. (NO, 1:298)

At the beginning of his discussion of the relationship between truth and utility Bacon acknowledges that the study of the material world, as opposed to the "contemplation of truth," is associated with anxiety, confusion, and falling, and with Tartarus. Tartarus is the dark region located as far beneath Hades as Hades is from heaven, the region most absent from light—a common metaphor in Bacon's work for spiritual and intellectual knowledge. The opposition between earth as a kind of nothingness and the fullness of divine truth is a dichotomy that supports the doctrine of *contemptus mundi* that powerfully condemns human efforts to investigate the material world. Though

Bacon's goal is to accomplish such an investigation, he follows a listing of the negative qualities traditionally attached to empirical study with "Now to this I readily assent." At this moment he links and separates himself from traditional doctrine. "This" is the voice of tradition; Bacon's submission to it seems to hazard his whole endeavor. His act of deference, however, elevates his project by allowing it to be inscribed within a metaphysical system. Once his project becomes traditional, tradition is transformed. While the symmetrical structure of the passage and Bacon's passive acquiescence lull us to sleep, Bacon performs a sleight of hand. The contemplation of truth is made equivalent to the study of the material world, which had earlier seemed the antithesis of it.

The "Ideas of the divine," Bacon tells us, can only be discovered by anatomizing the world. This claim gives his anatomical method the privileged status of an absolutely reliable means of interpretation. With such an instrument at his disposal, Bacon gains the authority to expose former philosophical systems as "Idols" and to replace them with the "true model" of science. He finishes by scattering old idols to the winds, thus dispersing the opposition to his new equation of truth and utility, theology and anatomy. Earlier anatomists inadvertently produced and discovered the decay of a traditional order—in the effort to cleanse the world by anatomizing it they expanded the domain of worthless matter. Bacon intends to recuperate the old order by the very means that decomposed it in the first place. He is optimistic where his predecessors are pessimistic because he has found a way to reconcile empirical techniques and the "Ideas of the divine"—or so he believes.

In spite of his shrewd analysis of the proclivity of men to establish insubstantial systems of order in place of truth, Bacon's own project was directed toward a utopia, a New Jerusalem.[5] It was important for the success of his ideas that this be so. The promise of absolute order helped subdue the fears of his audience about the consequence of a shift in the focus of knowledge from the contemplation of metaphysical truths to the contemplation of isolated facts that could not yet be placed within a formal system of knowledge. According to Bacon, "the fluctuations of individual things," the "turmoil and confusion" created by anatomizing matter, were not to be interpreted as signs of the decay of order, but as the precondition of its establishment. This new order was to be a genuine one, made of things themselves, not of empty words; it would be an order as ontologically secure as nature itself. Bacon locates it in a prelapsarian world where acts of language and knowledge are innocent, not yet separated from the truth of God and nature. This placement of his project insures that the anatomist will not create "apish images" of the world. His representations will be real, true, chaste, "the creator's own stamp upon creation." As Bacon explains it in the *Advancement,* the scientist imitates Adam's acts of knowledge, "the view of creatures and the imposition of names," innocent acts of knowledge because "As for the knowledge which induced the fall, it was . . . not the natural knowledge of creatures, but the moral knowledge of good and evil . . ." (A, 1:61). Those who were unwilling to relinquish an archaic system of knowledge, a reluctance that was understandable given the incompleteness of Bacon's system, were seen by Bacon as obstacles to the achievement of an order more absolute than the traditional order of microcosm and macrocosm. His mission was to attack the men and their idols that stood in the way of the absolute "Instauration" of order.

Bacon's strength, like that of earlier anatomists, lies less in the construction of a positive order than in the destruction of false ones.[6] In the manner of all anatomies, his treatises are based on the assumption that appearances have become detached from reality and that the anatomist must therefore cut through these fictions to get to the truth. Bacon's skill at dissection is demonstrated in his exposure of the fallacies of man and language in the doctrine of the idols. He treats idols, in one form or another, in almost all his works, because to reach the tangible and certain facts that lie at the foundation of knowledge, he has first to tear away the superstitious notions that hide the truth from sight.

The negative process of destroying idols has a seductive power, as do many violent gestures of beginning, because it appears to make possible a complete break with the stale and limiting traditions of the past. Since idols "make the world the bond-slave of human thought, and human thought the bond-slave of words" (NO, 1:274), their destruction promises to give men a new power to know and speak the truth. Yet in spite of Bacon's hopeful efforts to be a liberator of men, his project seems faced with insurmountable obstacles. By his own admission, the idols of the tribe, cave, and marketplace are all innate and presumably resistant to his attack. And there is a more serious difficulty with his fragmenting way to reach the truth. What would happen if the idols actually were destroyed? The idols of the tribe have their origins in the mind's tendency to presuppose that its perceptions can be trusted, and in the will and affections; the idols of the cave are caused by the effects of nature and nurture; the idols of the marketplace are the result of the distortion caused by the inevitable gap between words and things; the idols of the theater are compelling orders of words that men substitute for nature itself. The eradication of these idols would constitute an apocalyptic sweeping away of all that makes up human culture. To abolish error and construct a new order, Bacon is embarked on a program to abolish "man," as we know him.

Bacon insists that his forceful clearing away of received ideas is a precondition for the advancement of learning. Yet on closer inspection, Bacon's dissection of idols seems a ruthless, even murderous, activity rather than a therapeutic one. In *The Masculine Birth of Time,* for example, the scientist as anatomist proclaims both his hostility to the enemies of progress and the virtue of ruthlessness:

> It is bad luck for me that, for lack of men, I must compare myself with brute beasts. But when you have had time to reflect you will see things differently. You will admire beneath the veil of abuse the spirit that has animated my attack. You will observe the skill with which I have packed every word with meaning and the accuracy with which I have launched my shafts straight into their hidden sores.[7]

There are two ways of interpreting Bacon's comparison of himself with beasts in this manifestation of his enthusiasm for dismembering his opponents. He may have intended to say that as a lone man among beasts he cannot be compared with other men. This maneuver to separate himself from beasts has the effect of placing him in the category he wants to avoid. Or he may mean that because no other man has dared to be as ferociously direct as he, he seems to be a beast. In any case, inadvertently or not, he acknowledges the brute violence of his own techniques. He also points to the virtuosity of his dissection as a mark of his superiority to the men he pierces with his shafts. From a man who elsewhere claims he would have his doctrine "enter quietly into the minds that are fit and capable of receiving it" (NO, 1:263), the acts of negation on which his project depends seem unexpectedly harsh.

It is not only destruction of the old order but also the institution of the new one that receives a negative repressive emphasis by Bacon. Bacon's description of his project is couched in a rhetoric of imperialism. "And surely it would be disgraceful if, while the regions of the material globe,—that is, of the earth, of the sea, and of the stars,—have been in our times laid widely open and revealed, the intellectual globe should remain shut up within the narrow limits of old discoveries" (NO, 1:282). As explorers and colonizers anatomize the world, laying it open to master it, so Bacon will lay open the intellectual world. Such projects, as Timothy Reiss has pointed out, are often imaged as acts of sexual violence: the new scientist "is a conqueror enforcing his will, a man ravishing a woman. . . ."[8] Certainly, the act of vision described as an anatomizing process, to lay a body "widely open," suggests the violence and disruption involved in such acts of discovery. The conquering power of the eye cruelly violates the integrity of a body. Given the aggressiveness, the desire for dominance this language displays so forcefully, it is quite understandable that Bacon himself compares the anatomizing process of discovery to war.

The development of a military attitude toward the object of investigation is in fact one of the goals of Bacon's program to advance learning. No longer is learning to be an effeminate activity, a voluptuous playing with words. Instead, the man of knowledge will be an Alexander who uses his superior force to dominate space: "the arts which flourish in times while virtue is in growth, are military; and while virtue is in declination, are voluptuary" (A, 1:108). By restoring truth Bacon will restore the "fierceness of men's minds" (1:71). As in earlier anatomies, masculine rhetoric and logic are opposed to deceitful feminine forms or painted "idols." In what seems like an act of sexual aggression, the anatomist penetrates those idols to reveal their falseness and insubstantiality. This act of penetrating the idols that ensnare men produces, as he explains in *Valerius Terminus*, knowledge "for fruit or generation" while "Knowledge that tendeth but to satisfaction is but as a courtesan" (VT, 1:189).

Bacon recognizes that such acts of aggression can only be justified by his goal, the perfect restoration of knowledge, and fights against the tendency to make attacks on idols the end of his project rather than the means to an end. He deliberately separates himself from anatomists like Democritus, to whom he admits he is indebted, because the school of Democritus is "so busied with the particulars that it hardly attends to the structure" (NO, 1:269). When all structures are dissected and nothing put in their place, then men begin to despair. And despair, Bacon says elsewhere in the same work, is the greatest obstacle to the progress of science (1:286). His recognition of the dark side of the anatomizing process, the way it breeds despair about re-assembling a fragmented world, makes him turn from the demolition of idols to the task of enunciating the optimistic, utopian side of his project. As an antidote to despair, he offers hope: not as a positive norm (Bacon is too much the anatomist to manage that), but as a promise that the limits of the mind and language—limits he so persuasively describes—will one day be overcome. Bacon offers several reasons for his hope that progress can be made in human understanding, the most important of which is the method of induction itself.

In the traditional method of induction, a principle or opinion was shored up by supporting information rather than by being tested. Such a method cannot advance knowledge, and, according to Bacon, this proves its artificiality: "For what is founded on nature grows and increases; while what is founded on opinion varies but increases not" (NO, 1:274). For Bacon, nature becomes the external standard against which man-made methods are tested. His belief that he had found a "natural" scientific method to replace the method of enumeration, a belief that seems naive if the distortions of the mind and language are indeed innate, was nevertheless a powerful impetus to scientific studies. If a method could be found that was truly "natural" then men could transcend the limits of the idols and reestablish a perfect relation between perception and reality, words and things.

Bacon attempts to reinforce the "naturalness" of his method by establishing a correspondence between the stages of induction and what he says are the stages of human thinking: reception of sense data, classification of data, and finally interpretation of data.[9] But this correspondence between mind and method is misleading (an example of the mind's tendency to feign "correspondents and relations") not only because Bacon's definition of thinking is not substantiated but also because it disguises the fact that his method requires an assault on nature. The scientist who uses the method of induction must anatomize and distill objects in order to find the "forms" of nature, such qualities of matter as "dense, rare, hot, cold, heavy, light," that are supposed by Bacon to constitute an "alphabet" from which all natural compounds are made (DA, 1:469).[10] Forms are the basis of a perfect code of nature which, when made legible, will make nature totally comprehensible. The problem, as Bacon's practice shows, is that the endeavor to discover "forms" by anatomizing the world disrupts nature and generates a mass of contradictory information. In an attempt to control this information, Bacon provides a means of classification.

When Bacon searches for a form, he collects all the positive and negative instances of its occurrence and organizes them into "tables of discovery." As part of the process of discovering the form of heat, for example, he gives as a positive instance "The rays of the sun, especially in summer and at noon": as a negative instance, "The rays of the moon and of stars and comets are not found to be hot to the touch . . ." (NO, 1:308–9). Once all positive and negative instances are collected, the scientist simply eliminates contradictory instances until "there will remain at the bottom, all light opinions vanishing into smoke, a Form affirmative, solid and true and well-defined." The form of heat, then, should be a stable essence even if its outward attributes are relative and uncertain: "Heat, as far as regards the sense and touch of man, is a thing various and relative; insomuch that tepid water feels hot if the hand be cold, but cold if the hand be hot"

(1:320). Yet in spite of Bacon's promises, his process of discovery fails to conclude with the revelation of an affirmative form. The form of heat has neither form, nor visibility, nor tangibility. Bacon remarks: "For the heat and cold are not themselves perceptible to touch. . . . Nor . . . to the sight" (1:355). After removing "all ambiguity," he finds the form of heat is not a solid object but the ungraspable quality of "Motion."

Bacon believes motion is the form of heat because he has confidence in the efficacy of his tables of instances. In the characteristic manner of Bacon's writings, the tables are open structures that allow new information to be added and new conclusions to be made. Bacon's reliance on "tables of discovery" heralds a new age that replaced the traditional system of correspondences with a taxonomic system of order. According to Michel Foucalt, among the modifications in Western thought that resulted from this shift in modes of organizing is:

> the substitution of analysis for the hierarchy of analogies: in the sixteenth century, the fundamental supposition was that of a total system of correspondence (earth and sky, planets and faces, microcosm and macrocosm), and each particular similitude was then lodged within this overall relation. From now on, every resemblance must be subjected to proof by comparison, that is, it will not be accepted until its identity and the series of its differences have been discovered by means of measurement with a common unit, or, more radically, by its position in an order. . . . A complete enumeration will now be possible: whether in the form of an exhaustive census of all the elements constituting the envisaged whole, or in the form of a categorical arrangement that will articulate the field of study in its totality. . . .[11]

Bacon's treatises, unlike earlier, more rambling anatomies, attempt to provide a "categorical arrangement that will articulate the field of study in its totality," the field being nature itself. This is a herculean task, and Bacon's anatomizing technique for finding the basic elements of the natural order, a destructive rather than a constructive method of discovery, did not make it any easier to accomplish.

Bacon's emphasis on the negative instance, meant to insure impartial judgments, is an emphasis found in other anatomies, which, in proceeding by negatives, use a method that impedes the imposition of order. Bacon is an heir to this tradition, even though his work is born of a desire to bring all nature under control. His works are governed by antithesis, a rhetorical device that maintains the "whirl and eddy of argument" that Bacon both abhors and abets. In an excellent article on the strategies Bacon employs in the *Essays* to disrupt a reader's preconceptions, Stanley Fish has shown that the operation of antithesis encourages the reader to suspend conclusions in order to scrutinize all the contradictory information available on a subject.[12] Paoli Rossi also comments on Bacon's preoccupation with *antitheta* as a means to check the mind's tendency to jump to conclusions.[13] In both cases antithesis apparently advances the cause of Bacon's new science. But the use of antithesis as a strategy for maintaining an argument (NO, 1:545–57) may lead not to progress in knowledge but to paralysis, an endless play of oppositions. The structure of Lyly's antithetical *Anatomy of Wit* demonstrates the danger of Bacon's plan to "proceed at first by negatives, and at last to end in affirmatives" (1:320)— the process of negation endlessly postpones the arrival at synthesis. Many of Bacon's own works are a testament to the difficulty of reaching his goal, the final *Interpretation of Nature:* they are, by his own admission, fragments. Bacon's concern with the negative instance, with recording errors and cataloging monstrosities of nature, helped prove the incompleteness of existing explanations of nature, but that, of course, is not the same thing as providing a "true model of the world."

Bacon places a distance between his work and a rhetorical tour de force like Lyly's anatomy by attacking artificial systems of words and emphasizing the naturalness of his own project. He is attempting to create a science that "rests on the solid foundation of experience," which is unlike the literary sciences of the past that incline more "towards copie than weight" (A, 1:54). In accord with his commitment to focus on empirical reality, he rejects witty forms of discourse that are full of

words and far from nature itself. Bacon saw that the success of
his method to discover the "true model of the world" depended
on his ability to find a mode of communication that would
enable him to overcome the limits of the idols of the marketplace which impede attempts to represent the world as it
"really" is. The anatomy form encouraged the experiments in
style that Bacon conducted to create this new linguistic structure, as it had encouraged his critique of verbal structures. The
anatomist sets out to dissect the idols of language because he
suspects the integrity of words and this very suspicion compels
him to create new, and, one would hope, more legitimate, modes
of communication—euphuism, the exploded verbal universe
of Thomas Nashe, the aphoristic style of Sir Francis Bacon. All
three men are preoccupied with language, but whereas the styles
of Lyly and Nashe are self-consciously literary expressions of
reality, Bacon's is a style that effaces itself in an effort to become capable of representing truths external to language.

An examination of Bacon's aphoristic style, a paradigmatic
instance of the anatomical method, is useful for understanding
the aims, effects, and shortcomings of the aphorism as a mode
of scientific discourse. In the *Advancement,* Bacon says that
aphorisms "representing a knowledge broken, do invite men to
enquire farther, whereas Methods, carrying the shew of a total,
do secure men, as if they were at furthest" (A, 1:125). What
Bacon means by "Methods" is not his own inductive method
but traditional methods, such as the method of induction by
enumeration or the syllogism described in the *Novum Organum,*
which encourage acceptance rather than critical examination of
propositions. For example, of the syllogism he says:

> I . . . reject demonstration by syllogism, as acting too
> confusedly, and letting nature slip out of its hands. For
> although no one can doubt that things which agree in a
> middle term agree with one another (which is a proposi-
> tion of mathematical certainty), yet it leaves an opening
> for deception; which is this. The syllogism consists of
> propositions; propositions of words; and words are the
> tokens and signs of notions. Now if the very notions of the
> mind (which are as the soul of words and the basis of the

whole structure) be improperly and over-hastily abstracted from facts, vague, and not sufficiently definite, faulty in short in many ways, the whole edifice tumbles. (NO, 1:249)

Syllogistic logic is what Bacon calls a "magistral" method of communication that seduces the reader to accept as conclusions propositions that have never been proved. Magistral methods win consent because "they carry a kind of demonstration in orb or circle, one part illuminating another, and therefore satisfy . . ." (A, 1:125). In opposition to this method he proposes an "initiative" method, which, like the inductive method, is a procedure to make all the data on which a conclusion is based available to the readers so that they can examine them themselves and test any conclusions drawn from them. It emphasizes particulars to help the readers "suspend Judgement" until the data have been reviewed. The aphorisms of "ancient seekers after truth," recalls Bacon, presented knowledge in "short and scattered sentences, not linked together by an artificial method; and did not pretend or profess to embrace the entire art" (NO, 1:283).

This statement about aphorisms reveals the same desire to go outside rhetoric to nature that motivates Bacon's invention of the method of induction to replace the rhetorical method of enumeration. But though he here claims that aphorisms make it possible for nature to be represented naturally, other remarks show that he was self-conscious about the ways a fragmentary style persuades a reader of the validity of material an author presents. Lisa Jardine notes that Bacon himself discusses the way "unordered division of material gives the effect of profusion; ordered division adds the illusion that the coverage is complete, and the limits of investigation set."[14] She adds that Bacon favors aphorism because "unordered division also conveys the impression that there is further material to be investigated." Profusion and lack, these are the effects of aphorisitic style, independent of content. In *De Augmentis Scientiarum*, Bacon argues against the fallacy that "that which consists of many divisible parts is greater than that which consists of a few parts and is more one" (DA, 1:544) and later in the same work says "beware of fragments" (1:617). His critical dissection of the style of fragments is even more pronounced in *The Masculine Birth of Time,* in which he attacks the wisdom of Hippocrates conveyed in aphorisms. Hippocrates, he says, protects himself from scrutiny "according to the fashion of his age by an oracular brevity. . . . But in truth the oracle is dumb. He utters nothing but a few sophisms sheltered from correction by their curt ambiguity. . . ."[15] These shrewd objections to the aphoristic method make readers more confident in Bacon's ability to avoid the snares of aphorisms when he uses them himself. After all, his aphorisms, unlike those of Hippocrates, are apparently uncompromised by an artificial linguistic arrangement.

But it is Bacon's recognition that language is always an artificial order that compels his persistent efforts to avoid it. In fact, a mistrust of even mathematical languages encouraged him to develop a system of investigation, the inductive method, that appears to begin from scratch. His use of aphorisms was also designed to reduce language to a minimum in order to bring the content of a proposition to a maximum. In other words, he reduces both nature and language so language will seem unobtrusive and nature undeniably present. But as Bacon's own objections to what he calls "ridiculous" aphorisms show, there is no reason to assume that the content and value of a proposition will increase if the number of words it contains is as small as possible (A, 1:125). The very compactness of aphorisms may instead make them enigmatic or "oracular" rather than clear and straightforward.

Bacon admits he values a veiled method of communication in his studies of fables and parables but he does not comment on the hieroglyphic character of his own aphorisms. He does say that nature is a labyrinth, and, since he says often that his method mirrors nature, we may take this as a warning. Aphorisms are like hieroglyphs because they are dark, "oracular" forms that, like nature itself, must be anatomized if their hidden meaning is to be revealed. They are also a similitude, a visual hieroglyph, of the particulars of nature. Hieroglyphs, as Bacon notes, both hide meaning and reveal it (DA, 1:441). An aphorism demands dissection as a way to reveal its hidden truth; but it also is supposed to represent the solid kernel of fact that remains after a dissection has been made. Its contradictory message is another hieroglyph, a sign of Bacon's transitional position between traditional and modern styles of knowledge. The aphorism is the zero point where science and alchemy come together—it not only makes nature present, it also defers that presencing by veiling nature. This veiled form entices the reader to participate with Bacon in an alchemical delving into the mysteries of nature. The "pith and heart of the sciences" is also the philosopher's stone of the alchemist.

As we have seen, these two sides of Bacon's science are evident not only in the aphorism but also in the negative instance that allows and postpones the discovery of an affirmative form, and in the use of antithesis to prevent the mind from jumping to false conclusions, or arriving at true ones. This doubleness, though it impedes construction of the "true model" of science, gives his project rhetorical force. The man who uses Bacon's methods has the power to dispel illusion and to create the illusion, the dream, of a future in which mute objects will speak truths that will make all things possible. These two poles of his project, scientific and alchemical, justify science and inspire faith in its telos.

Faith that an "anatomy of the world" will lead to "utility and fruit" links Bacon's method to power as well as truth. Earlier anatomists had complained that knowledge was severed from power. Lyly and Nashe, for example, suffered from a sense that learning was not valued by society and this prompted them to attack their own education as well as the people in power who neglected learned men like them. The estrangement of the anatomists is marked by their anatomies: Euphues goes into exile; Nashe's anatomist is an alienated, discontented scholar. But Bacon places the man who anatomizes tradition at the heart of society, a place perhaps equivalent to his own as Lord Chancellor of England. As Reiss notes, the power of Bacon's own voice demonstrates "the developing of analytico-referential dominance."[16] Anatomy, one of the primary modes of this discourse, is now endowed with the capacity to control the wealth of nature. The new anatomist is a figure of magnificence as Bacon's description of the scientist in the *New Atlantis* shows:

He was a man of middle stature and age, comely of person, and had an aspect as if he pitied men. He was clothed in a robe of fine black cloth, with wide sleeves and a cape. His garment was of excellent white linen down to the foot, girt with a girdle of the same; and a sindon or tippet of the same about his neck. He had gloves that were curious, and set with stone; and shoes of peach-colored velvet. . . . He was carried in a rich chariot without wheels litter-wise; with two horses at either end, richly trapped in blue velvet embroidered, and two footmen on each side in like attire. The chariot was all of cedar, gilt, and adorned with crystal; save the fore-end had pannel of sapphires, set in borders of gold, and the hinder-end the like of emeralds of the Peru color. (*New Atlantis*, 3:154–55)

His knowledge, symbolized by a "sun of gold radiant upon the top," dazzles as much as his possessions do. One depends on the other. The scientist is given wealth because his knowledge is valuable, his knowledge leads to the production of the wealth he is given in payment. No one begrudges him absolute rule. The future—political, economic, linguistic—lies with the man who adopts the anatomical techniques promoted by Bacon.

The visage of the "Father of Saloman" suggests, though, that his eminence exacts a cost: he has an "aspect as if he pitied men." The importance of method is only comprehensible if one grasps the limits of human intelligence and the necessity of "helps." As Bacon says, "if I have made any progress, the way has been opened to me by no other than the true and legitimate humiliation of the human spirit" (NO, 1:246). In order to find the lucrative truth of nature, one must paradoxically accept the estrangement of human perception and language from nature. Earlier anatomists had separated themselves from society, but the separation is now internalized, the intellect is separated from nature rather than the individual from society. This estrangement marks the shift from the order of microcosm and macrocosm to the order of taxonomy. The mistrust of apparent resemblances between the world of man and of nature, words and things, led to the proliferation of anatomies that cut through appearances, breaking objects down into the simplest elements, which were then rearranged in a taxonomic order quite different from the apparent order of the world that had once been so full of significance. The cost of this shift, as Reiss puts it, was not only a loss of "confidence in Man's energies, in his capacity to seize and conduct the world around him in his own name," but even more "the revelation of the insufficiencies of our sense impressions and of the impossibility of our basing any intellectual systems of the external world upon them. A contract between mind and matter was lost. Man placed himself to one side of matter."[17] That break between mind and matter, language and nature, could not be bridged within language itself, even the carefully formed language structures of Bacon's new science.

The ending of the old and the beginning of a new relation between man and language is the subject of Hugo von Hofmannsthal's "The Letter of Lord Chandos." The letter, supposedly from Lord Chandos, an English gentleman, to Bacon, is written to explain why Lord Chandos will never write again. The implications of the doctrine of the idols have overwhelmed him. Lord Chandos had once been a passionate man of letters, a man much like Bacon himself, who wrote plays, pastorals, and Latin treatises, and entertained plans to write a history of Henry VIII, to decipher the fables of the ancients, to write an encyclopedic book unlocking the mysteries of nature:

> To sum up: In those days I, in a state of continuous intoxication, conceived the whole of existence as one great unit: the spiritual and the physical worlds seemed to form no contrast, as little as did courtly and bestial conduct, art and barbarism, solitude and society; in everything I felt the presence of Nature, in the aberrations of insanity as much as in the utmost refinement of the Spanish ceremonial; in the boorishness of young peasants no less than in the most delicate of allegories; and in all expressions of Nature I felt myself. When in my hunting lodge I drank the warm foaming milk which an unkempt wench had drained into a wooden pail from the udder of a beautiful gentle-eyed cow, the sensation was no different from that which I experienced when, seated on a bench built into the window of my study, my mind absorbed the sweet foaming nourish-

ment from a book. The one was like the other, . . . whether
in dreamlike celestial quality or in physical intensity—and
thus it prevailed through the whole expanse of life in all
directions; everywhere I was in the centre of it, never sus-
pecting mere appearance. . . .

His use of the past tense indicates that appearances have become
suspect. A sense that words are separate from the presence of
nature compels him to look more closely at language and the
men that use it: he conducts an anatomy. But here anatomy is
not a construct with positivity: "For me everything disintegrated
into parts, those parts again into parts; no longer would anything let itself be encompassed by one idea."[18] Occasionally
Lord Chandos could find consolation in natural images of isolation and entrapment—a crippled person, rats locked in a poi-
soned cellar—that linked him again to the external world.
Finally he decided that to reappropriate presence he must
eschew all forms of mediation: Lord Chandos embraces silence.

One can imagine Bacon, after reading this letter, composing
a note to his friend prescribing the ministrations of his method
as the means to overcome the inadequacy of words. He could
remain calm in the face of anxiety generated from his own
doctrines because his dream of order protected him from the
knowledge that anatomizing nature might destroy it, or the
possibility that anatomizing opened up a problematic relation
between words and things that would compromise his own work
as well as that of the ancients. Bacon was more right than he
knew when he speculated that future generations would say of
him what a Roman historian had said of Alexander: "All
Alexander did was dare to despise shams."[19] Bacon despised the
false orders that serve for our reality but could not replace them
with "real" ones. What he bequeathed to the centuries that followed was an insatiable desire to enclose nature and an anatomizing method that was both the means and the obstacle to
satisfying that desire. Modern science, and the disciplines it has
sponsored, are heirs to the satisfactions and frustrations of
Bacon's desire and his methods.

7 · *Anatomy as Reason and Madness*

COMPARED WITH BACON'S dynamic, scientific project to inaugurate a new order of things, Burton's great lumpy *Anatomy of Melancholy* looks particularly hesitant and unfocused. And because of this, Burton's work serves as a reminder that the institution of "analytico-referential" discourse did not end all questions about the proper way to get at the truth. *The Anatomy of Melancholy* is narrated by an "I" that worries about its madness rather than by a persona confident of its powers—and this "I" is madly ambivalent about its own anatomical practice. As a result, *The Anatomy of Melancholy* seems both a return to older, marginal anatomies and a harbinger of our own moment of epistemological uncertainty. I don't want to suggest that Burton is simply a protodeconstructionist but rather that Burton's *Anatomy* helps complicate our sense of history as a progress from one discourse to the next by *failing* to exemplify the growing dominance of analytical discourse in the seventeenth century. We are particularly able to sympathize with this failing, I think, because of our own uncertainties about how writing constitutes the truth of God, nature, and the self.

Robert Burton's *Anatomy of Melancholy,* the best known example of the Renaissance anatomy, is the last instance of the anatomy as an immensely popular literary mode. It is also the last anatomy of the period that self-consciously exhibits the paradoxes of the form. The Renaissance anatomy certainly gives rise to the anatomies written in the Age of Reason, but it lacks the single-minded attachment to the discourse of rationalism that characterizes most of them. Yet that discourse fathered by Bacon has so influenced our own thinking that it is difficult not to defend Burton's *Anatomy* by suggesting that it meets criteria for literary excellence—the work's truth to life, its organic unity—established in the eighteenth century. One critic, for example, writes that Burton uses the "method of anatomy because it enables him to unify the diversity of human knowledge and reduce madness to method."[1] This statement raises hope that Burton, even more than Bacon, will satisfy a reader's desire for a unified and clear meaning. Perhaps Burton, unlike other anatomists, has a godlike ability to organize "human knowledge" and perform the difficult trick of turning madness into reason. Certainly the *Anatomy of Melancholy,* with its elaborate scholarly apparatus, attempts to give the reader an orderly account of an unruly subject, melancholy madness. But how do we reconcile the scholarly strategies of the *Anatomy* with Burton's swirling, disorderly prose?

A possible reconciliation is inherent in Burton's chosen mode of writing: an anatomy will reduce a body to order by turning it into a heap of fragments. The strength of the *Anatomy* lies in this paradox. Animated by a struggle between reason and madness, order and fragmentation, Burton's text demonstrates its power not by imposing order, but by escaping all efforts to have an order imposed on it. *Anatomy of Melancholy* is located on the boundary that lies between reason and madness. It is a scientific and theological treatise—and a mirror of the madness that is the book's subject. No wonder, then, that critics have found it difficult to classify Burton's text.[2] The titles and subtitles of critical commentaries—*Sanity in Bedlam; The Tangled Chain: The Structure of Disorder in the Anatomy of Melancholy; "The Anatomy of Melancholy:* Confusion and Order" (the central subheading of an article)—record the coexistence of two antagonists, reason and madness, in the same text.[3]

Yet the full title of Burton's life work, *The Anatomy of Melancholy What it is, with all the kinds, causes, symptomes, prognostickes & severall cures of it,* is not an announcement of textual ambiguity. Instead, the title prepares us for a comprehensive medical study, perhaps the sort of book one physician has claimed it to be: "a great medical treatise, orderly in arrangement, serious in purpose, and weighty beyond belief with authorities."[4] Burton's concern with medical material, his provision of synoptic tables, copious footnotes, and an index all do suggest rigorous order. Certainly the work is serious in purpose. Like other anatomists, Burton has a commitment to revealing the truth that lies at the heart of things; and, as a divine as well as an anatomist, he has a double commitment to the revealed truth. There are good reasons to believe that *Anatomy of Melancholy* is a comprehensive work of knowledge.

Burton even sounds like Bacon when he announces his goals. In the opening section, he says he will "perspicuously define what this melancholy is, show his name and differences" (1.1.169).[5] This labor is justified by its usefulness: Burton will make melancholy "more familiar and easy for every man's capacity, and the common good, which is the chief end of my discourse" (1.1.139). A rigorous anatomical analysis is for the "common good" because it leads to the recovery of absolute truth as it cures madness. In the preface, Burton imagines an anatomizing orderer who is able to "root out barbarism," "cut off our tumultuous desires," "root out atheism, impiety, heresy, schism, and superstition," though Burton takes a milder course (P, 97). He will cure madness by subjecting it to a structure of reason. If madness is the condition that has beset all men since the Fall, reason should be able to cure it. Such a cure is of unusual importance: "I know not wherein to do a more general service . . . than to prescribe means how to prevent and cure so universal a malady" (120–21). An anatomy of melancholy will undo one of the gravest consequences of the Fall, man's loss of perfect reason. Perhaps even more than Bacon, Burton insists on the power of his fragmenting technique to restore wholeness: his anatomy will restore human reason so that all will know the original truth.

As we saw in Bacon's work, a commitment to recovering the naked truth by conducting an anatomy requires a new kind of language. Burton too announces that he has adopted a style in which words will be subordinate to matter:

I am *aquae potor* [a water-drinker], drink no wine at all, which so much improves our modern wits, a loose, plain, rude writer, *ficum voco ficum et ligonem ligonem* [I call a fig a fig and a spade a spade], and as free, as loose, *idem calamo quod in mente* [what my mind thinks my pen writes], I call a spade a spade, *animis haec scribo, non auribus* [I write for the mind, not the ear], I respect matter, not words; remembering that of Cardan, *verba propter res, non res propter verba* [words should minister to matter, not vice versa], and seeking with Seneca, *squid scribam, non quemadmodum,* rather what than how to write: for as Philo thinks, "He that is conversant about matter neglects words, and those that excel in this art of speaking have no profound learning." (P, 31–32)

To call "a spade a spade" is in accord with Burton's project to get at the truth through the process of anatomy: "I will adventure to guess as near as I can, and rip them [the causes of melancholy] all up, from the first to the last, general and particular" (1.2.177–78). With zeal characteristic of the anatomist, Burton will rip up the truth and present it without embellishment; he wants to discover a true model of a universal disease, melancholy.

Burton announces that his is a plain style, tells us his intention to cure disease, gives his text a scholarly form; so a reader expects the *Anatomy* to be clear, useful, orderly. Yet Burton himself questions this view of his text. His assertion that he will provide a complete description of melancholy is deeply qualified. Burton will "adventure" to "guess as near as he can" about the causes of this madness. A guess does not have the authority of one of Bacon's forms, "solid, and true and well-defined." Furthermore, Burton's protestation against words is excessively wordy. He may repeat the claims of scientific discourse to a "naturalness" that allows it to represent things without the interference of words, but when we read the text what we notice are the words the "plain style" means to efface. Finally, the Baconian hope for anatomy as a method of restoring a "whole" truth, whether of nature, man, or God, cannot be sustained. Indeed, it occurs to Burton that the very desire for the "whole" truth might be a symptom of madness: "To insist in all particulars were an Herculean task, to reckon up *insanas substructiones, insanos labores, insanum luxum,* mad labours, mad books, endeavours, carriages, gross ignorance, ridiculous actions, absurd gestures . . ." (P, 116–17). Says Jean Starobinski: "Ce clergyman mélancholique a parfaitement démontré l'aspect désespérant et désespéré de tout ce qui s'est appelé science jusqu'à ce jour: à force de sagesse accumulée et juxtaposée, il a rendu manifeste une secrète folie."[6] Burton exposes the madness of the desire to represent the truth, even as he adopts the strategy of anatomy precisely because he believes it is a pathway to truth.

The tension between Burton's belief in reason and his suspicion of its limits exists even in the first partition, the most scientific section of the *Anatomy,* which gives the reader reason to doubt the very possibility of reason. The section begins with a discussion of "Man's Excellency, Fall, Miseries, Infirmities, the causes of them." Man has been separated from the truth as a result of the Fall and, according to the words of the Bible, this original transgression is punished by God with yet more "madness, blindness, and astonishing of heart" (1.1.132). The body too is an obstacle to rational understanding: man is "bad by nature" (1.1.136). And this is not all that interferes with the ability to see things clearly. In the "Digression of Spirits" which follows, devils, witches, and magicians also assault the minds of men. Confusion, it seems, is man's inheritance.

The mind is blinded, the body corrupt, and "dwelling" between the confines of sense and reason are "pertubations and passions" (1.2.258). Whether passions and pertubations are initiated by the mind (the soul's effort to "smite the body") or by the body ("they follow sense more than reason"), they seem to mark the place where the body and mind meet and interfere with each other. The passions disorder the already disorderly realms of matter and mind with the help of the major instrument of the passions, the imagination.

The imagination is a faculty that causes the confusion of fiction and fact. Burton tells stories of those whose imaginations have turned illusions into reality:

> that melancholy men and sick men conceive so many phantastical visions, apparitions to themselves, and have such absurd suppositions, as that they are kings, lords, cocks,

bears, apes, owls; that they are heavy, light, transparent, great and little, senseless and dead. . . . can be imputed to naught else but to a corrupt, false, and violent imagination. It works not only in sick and melancholy men only, but even most forcibly sometimes in such as are sound. . . . And sometimes a strong conceit or apprehension, as Valesius proves, will take away diseases: in both kinds it will produce real effects. (1:2:255)

In this remarkable passage, Burton tells us that reality may be a product of the imagination. The imaginations of both the sane and the insane have "real effects." A reality built of the projections of the mind is always shifting: it is the play of transformation that Burton attempts to articulate by naming the multiple and contradictory roles that comprise the unstable "reality" of men. But Burton's discourse, however long-winded, is never long enough to describe them all, for as a result of the workings of the imagination, "reality" is always in flux and cannot be fully articulated.

As we have seen in earlier chapters, anatomy causes confusions similar to those Burton attributes to the workings of the imagination. As an anatomy empties out a body in order to make its hidden content visible, those contents are turned into surfaces, images, appearances. Anatomy, then, may itself be a cause of the "shipwreck of reason." Yet paradoxically, the failure of anatomy to discover a stable truth is a key to the success of Burton's work. Because the anatomy is a process of ordering that discovers disorder, it is a method suited to uncovering the disorderly nature of madness, though not to curing it.

The nature of melancholy is to elude all order. Even the simple classificatory scheme of the theory of humors used to isolate melancholy and place it in a rational order does not work for Burton (traditionally, melancholy is one of the four humors, coldness and dryness are its major qualities, and its primary seat is in the spleen). He tells his readers that melancholy may be "hot, cold, dry, moist" (1.3.399) and "no physician can truly say what part is affected" (1.3.411). Its causes cannot be classified ("there is no one cause of this melancholy humor") nor can its symptoms:

> Who can sufficiently speak of these symptoms, or prescribe
> rules to comprehend them? . . . The four-and-twenty let-
> ters make no more variety of words in divers languages
> than melancholy conceits produce diversity of symptoms in
> several persons. They are irregular, obscure, various, so in-
> finite, Proteus himself is not so diverse; you may as well
> make the moon a new coat as a true character of a melan-
> choly man; as soon find the motion of a bird in the air as
> the heart of man, a melancholy man. . . . Who can dis-
> tinguish these melancholy symptoms so intermixed with
> others, or apply them to their several kinds, confine them
> into method? 'Tis hard, I confess; yet I have disposed of
> them as I could, and will descend to particularize them
> according to their species. (1.3.408)

Burton's long *apologia* tells us that the nature of melancholy
escapes classification. Melancholy is determined to remain mad
in spite of all efforts to "confine" it "into a method" and make
it obey reason.

Burton's discussion of the humors reveals his awareness of
the failure of rational schemes to adequately represent the object
of his study, melancholy. The theory of humors, as he shows, is
not able to make melancholy perfectly intelligible; there is a
gap between the theory and what it represents. And when we
look at Burton's synoptic tables and compare them to his
sprawling text, we feel a similar disjunction between a referent,
here the text, and a representation of it, the synopses. Certainly
the tables indicate Burton's interest in making his text appear
coherent and well planned, and readers who share this desire
tend to see the tables as the center, a kind of "skeleton," of the
text.[7] These readers who privilege the tables over the text are
optimistic anatomists. But the order of the synoptic tables is a
kind of mask that not only hides but also gives rise to the disorder so basic to the anatomy form.

At first glance the tables appear to provide a clear picture of
the text. David Renaker, one of Burton's most perceptive critics,
says that "a close comparison of these charts with the text shows
that they are not mere mystification; they are a map of the
book."[8] Nonetheless, there is a great difference between the

order of a map and the complex windings of Burton's narration. One reason for the clarity of the map is its clear spatial organization. Anatomists, of course, have an attachment to spatial models—the process of anatomy is meant to reduce a body into discrete parts that can be placed within the order of an anatomical table or chart. In this instance, the tables provide a spatial representation of the body of Burton's narration, which is a temporal discourse. And Burton's narration is protracted—each new edition is different from the one that precedes it—whereas from edition to edition the tables never change. In some sense, then, the tables lend the text a false simplicity and coherence.

Burton seems to have realized that his tables had the power to provide his text with the appearance of order, no matter how complicated a maze of details, anecdotes, and paradoxes his text became. Renaker shows that the logic of the tables seems to give Burton license to indulge his fascination with all the divergent ways that melancholy manifests itself. Because of the solidity of the tables, Burton "felt free to regard each part of his world, for the moment he was treating it, as an absolute, ignoring or forgetting its relation to the others."[9] He uses the same information to prove opposite points, an illogical practice, while trusting the tables to provide an overall logic. The tables, then, do their job too well.

Burton's contradictory text thus diverges from the orderly tables. Yet, remembering that in the process of anatomy the inside becomes the outside, we might expect to find something of the text's ambiguities in the tables that frame it. And they are there. The tables do not so much provide a picture of order as a picture of the difficulties an anatomist has in creating coherence through a process of fragmentation. When we look at the tables, we see that subsections proliferate and entries that cannot contain their subjects end with "etc." To the extent that the tables do mirror the text, they participate in its disorder.

Burton's numerous citations are also symptoms of the interplay of order and disorder characteristic of the anatomy. The citations found in the text and in its margins advertise it as scholarly and well ordered. References, after all, are normally used to establish that an author has carefully researched a topic and has taken pains to use source material so as to neither falsely appropriate it nor distort it. Yet Burton's references are anything but an assurance that he values a truthful representation of other texts: instead of carefully repeating the words of others, he actively manipulates them. David Renaker has recorded the transformation that one name, Cleombrotus of Ambracia, goes through when Burton cites it. The result of his investigation gives proof that Burton's scholarship is similar to Nashe's linguistic play: Cleombrotus of Ambracia becomes "Theombrotus Ambrociato," "Theombrotus Ambraciotes," and "Cleombrotus Amborciatus."[10] Burton's quotations are often inventions, and what seems his own invention is sometimes a quotation. F. P. Wilson has discovered a passage from what is supposedly Burton's prose that is in fact an "almost verbatim" quotation from another text.[11] Like the tables, the notes provide an assurance of order while contributing to disorder.

Burton is not always comfortable with using quotations as a means of appropriating the words of others. Sounding much like Nashe, Burton complains about "pilfering" writers who dissect old texts: "they pilfer out of old writers to stuff up their new comments, scrape Ennius' dung-hills, and out of Democritus' pit, as I have done. By which means it comes to pass, 'that not only libraries and shops are full of our putrid papers, but every close-stool and jakes'" (P, 23). Yet later he cheerfully admits that his text is "all mine and none mine" (P, 24). The announcement reflects his belief that texts inevitably undergo a transformation when placed in new contexts:

> The matter is theirs most part, and yet mine, *apparet unde sumptum sit* [it is plain whence it was taken] (which Seneca approves), *aliud tamen quam unde sumptum sit apparet,* [yet it becomes something different in its new setting]. . . . I must usurp that of Wecker *e Ter., nihil dictum quod non dictum prius, methodus sola artificem ostendit,* we can say nothing but what hath been said. . . .
> (P, 25)

Here Burton discusses and demonstrates how old texts gain a new life by being assimilated into new ones: what he "usurps" sounds as if it is his own. Apparently the anatomizing practice of ripping pieces of texts from their context may be either a means of fertilizing a text or a way of signifying a decay of invention. Quotation in Burton's text is both fertile and sterile. At times, particularly in the first partition, the text is a lifeless repetition of what has already been said. But, for the most part, in repeating and restating, Burton creates a distinctive mode of writing: a particular style of excessive quotation is recognizably his.

Fragments of texts provide the not very solid foundation of the *Anatomy,* and from this learned debris Burton digresses. He moves from the texts of other writers ever deeper into the realm of displaced representation; digression constitutes a breaking off from what has already been broken off. No wonder that it is not always easy to tell the difference between Burton's quotations and his own prose, or to establish the beginnings and ends of his narrative detours. In the "Digression of Air," Burton makes a connection between the flights away from his own material and the diving, probing process of anatomy: "But hoo! I am now gone quite out of sight, I am almost giddy with roving about: I could have ranged farther yet, but I am an infant, and not able to dive into these profundities or sound these depths, not able to understand, much less to discuss" (2.2.60). The "Digression of Air" begins with Burton's famous comparison of his progress of discovery to the flight of a "long-winged hawk." This is a happy metaphor of a voyage free from any secure ground: even if he is almost "giddy," the voyager enjoys that freedom. The passage also tells us that the hawk's flight *from* is also a dive *into* matter. Burton's metaphor, then, acknowledges the circularity of his investigative strategy—and its inevitable failure to arrive at any fundamentals, any "profundities." Instead, Burton's groundless text circles and repeats.

A world in which everything is dislocated from the ground of its meaning is a mad world. Stanley Fish remarks in exasperation: "nothing . . . can maintain its integrity in the context of an all-embracing madness. . . . Even syntactical and rhetorical forms—sentences, paragraphs, sections—lose their firmness in this most powerful of all solvents."[12] Fish blames madness for the condition of Burton's prose, but perhaps method is to blame, for the means that Burton uses to control madness, anatomy, is itself a kind of solvent. Instead of curing madness, Burton's *Anatomy* seems to create it. And if Burton's discourse is mad, how do we separate the object of investigation from the language that presents it to us?

By turning madness into language, a process of externalization basic to anatomy, language is turned more and more into madness—a condition it apparently has long participated in. Burton compares the "chaos of melancholy" to the effects of the Tower of Babel (1.3.397) and remarks that madness takes as many forms as the "variety of words" made by "four and twenty letters" (1.3.408). Once the original unity of words and referents is lost, words multiply, transform, and become impediments to meaning. To find a man who is not mad, Burton suggests we look for one who is silent: *"vir sapit qui pauca loquitur* [he is a wise man who says little]: no better way to avoid folly and madness than by taciturnity" (P, 117–18).

Bacon tries to tame the swirling world of words by adopting an aphoristic style that requires as few of them as possible, but Burton's technique generates more and more words: with each new edition the *Anatomy* grows. It grows because Burton believes that knowledge comes from the books he quotes even though he also fears that too much learning may lead to madness. His pride in his scholarship is tempered by his sense that learned men are creators of and sufferers of madness: "Bale, Erasmus, Hospinian, Vives, Kemnisius, explode as a vast ocean of *obs* and *sols,* school divinity. A labyrinth of intricable questions, and unprofitable contentions, *incredibilem delirationem* [an incredible doting] one calls it. . . . Much learning *cere-diminuit-brum,* hath cracked their sconce" (P, 111–12). He also calls learned men "crazy rhetoricians," "note-makers," and other terms that point to their verbosity. But even as he exposes these scribblers, Burton keeps on writing. In the process of cutting through false words, he generates more surface, more debris, more madness.

As with Nashe's literary criticism, the works Burton anatomizes reflect characteristics of his own work. Since Burton says that a book full of "intricable questions" is a symptom of a "cracked sconce," we might suspect that Burton's head was also cracked. Joan Webber and other critics have noted that the *Anatomy* is a kind of mirror of Burton's mind, which as Burton tells us is pained by a "kind of imposthume" called melancholy (P, 21).[13] In anatomical terms, we could say that Burton's mind is the "inside" substance that is externalized through the process of anatomy. Burton uses metaphors of the theater to describe the externalized condition of the self: "I have put myself upon the stage" (P, 27). This condition is apparently universal: "he, and he, and he, and the rest are all hypocrites, ambidexters, outsides, so many turning pictures" (P, 65). Because of the operation of anatomy, or perhaps because the world itself is mad, the self lacks a secure foundation.

Burton took pains to insure that the "I" of his narration was an "outside" or "turning picture," as the development of the *Anatomy* shows.[14] In the first edition Burton makes an effort to anchor his "I" to his own name: he attaches a conclusion in which he takes off the mask of Democritus that he has put on in the preface. "The last section shall be more to cut the strings of Democritus visor, to unmaske and shew him as he is." The unmasking takes the form of a signature that ends the book: "From my Studie in Christ-Church Oxon—Robert Burton."[15] In the first edition, then, the text seems to move from the veiled "I" of the preface to the unveiled "I" of the conclusion, a kind of revelation that seems compatible with the act of anatomy as a process that cuts through false appearances and brings the truth to light. In later editions, however, Burton deliberately frustrates the equation of author and persona, dropping the conclusion and adding a frontispiece in which he includes a picture of himself. This picture offers assurance that we will find the real Burton inside the text, but the text turns this apparently unified identity (but an identity that is only an "outside") into a series of yet other masks. From the clarity of the picture, we move into a discourse in which the "I" of the narrator is never given the stability of Burton's name.

Although the narrator does claim a proper name for himself, "Democritus Junior," this does not secure the narrator's identity, for, as Stanley Fish has pointed out, "we have as many Democrituses as we have sources for his life, and not all of them are compatible."[16] However, the *Anatomy* gains by this instability.

The mask of Democritus allows the narrator "to assume a little more liberty and freedom of speech" (P, 19). The excesses of the voice Burton adopts, its violence and liberties, are spoken by "another person":

> If I have overshot myself in this which hath been hitherto said, or that it is, which I am sure some will object, too phantastical, "too light and comical for a divine, too satirical for one of my profession," I will presume to answer, with Erasmus in like case, 'Tis not I, but Democritus, *Democritus dixit:* you must consider what it is to speak in one's own or another's person, an assumed habit and a name. . . . (P, 121)

" 'Tis not I, but Democritus"—Who is speaking here? The "I" is clearly different from Democritus, though Democritus is also a replacement for it. If the "I" is Robert Burton, it is Robert Burton as an "outside" created by anatomy: "I have . . . in this treatise . . . turned my inside outward" (P, 27). But the confusion caused by the process of turning an inside outward makes it difficult to separate outside mask and inside self.

The same problems arise when we try to separate the preface from the "serious" content of the *Anatomy,* as some critics have done. The preface incorporates parts of the conclusion that Burton discarded after the first edition, which makes the preface simultaneously a beginning and an ending. It is based on "inside" content—a conclusion follows from the reading of a text—and yet seems to stand "outside" the text as a point of entry. Once again, inside and outside merge. And does the reader remain safely outside this troublesome discourse? The narrator tells the reader: "Thou thyself art the subject of my discourse" (P, 16). With these words, the reader is pulled inside the text and the reader's interior is made into something external. Such maneuvers exacerbate the problems caused by anatomy—and lead us into madness.

This madness is apparently inescapable because "we are all mad" (P, 71). In the second edition Burton finds only one exception to this general condition, and that exception is "Nemo":

Nemo; nam, Nemo omnibus horis sapit, Nemo nascitur sine vitiis, Crimine Nemo caret, Nemo sorte sua vivit contentus, Nemo in amore sapit, Nemo bonus, Nemo sapiens, Nemo est ex omni parti beatus [Nobody; for Nobody is sensible at all times; Nobody is born without fault; Nobody is free from blame; Nobody lives content with his own lot; Nobody is sane in love; Nobody is good, Nobody wise, Nobody is completely happy], etc. (P, 117)

When the anatomist gets to the truth, nothing is left. Nobody is fit to reside in Burton's utopia, the nowhere in which life is properly ordered. If the mad world of man is without substance, so is the one the anatomist hopes to discover through his anatomical cure of melancholy.

Adrift without anchor, the melancholy mind is conventionally depicted to be "at sea."[17] Michel Foucault notes that melancholy, "la maladie anglaise," was believed to result from the influence of a maritime climate which could make the mind lose its firmness. English freedom was also proposed as a cause for melancholy because freedom leaves men uncertain about what to believe: "the penalty of liberty" is "indecision" and an "irresolute attention, of the vacillating soul."[18] The vacillation that is so much a part of Burton's *Anatomy* leads finally to despair. In the final section, Burton writes about despairing men who are "tossed in a sea, and that continually without rest or intermission" (3.4.405). The *Anatomy* that begins as a voyage to discover an original truth arrives at despair about the existence of such a truth. Of course, this despair also vacillates. Burton's closing command offers solace: SPERATE MISERI [Hope, ye unhappy ones], before taking it away: CAVETE FELICES [ye happy ones, fear]. If Burton's text leads to despair and frustration because it goes nowhere, it is also engagingly dedicated to journey, to endless promise. What is surprising is that there was such a large audience for this kind of narrative, such a shared sense of the uncertainty at the foundation of things. This uncertainty made necessary and enjoyable a flood of words not subservient to any clear pattern of meaning.

Does Burton's *Anatomy* reveal the human condition in the country from which the French name the disease? Or does he simply project his own condition on others? Critics have written about the *Anatomy* as a document of social and economic change that reflects the rise of scientific rationalism that threw all in doubt. Others have pointed out that Burton's text reveals his own uncertain position as scholar and divine.[19] Mueller, for one, writes that scholars were often poor, jobless, and lonely. In the "Digression of the Misery of Scholars and why the Muses are Melancholy," Burton writes that scholars "striving to be excellent lose health, wealth, wit, life, and all" (1.2.306). They lose all because they are neglected by patrons and because their labors often produce no fruit. Like Lyly and Nashe, Burton was a displaced and marginal man whose anatomy offers a critique of the society that could not offer him a better place. Yet Burton, equivocal as always, wonders if the scholar's exile from the domain of power might not be deserved: what seems to be the striving for excellence in the service of others might be only the fruitless activity of a mind turned in on itself. His uncertainty about whom to blame for his condition, and the condition of those like him, blunts the force of the *Anatomy* as social criticism—though given the vacillating nature of the melancholiac and the plethora of contradictory information turned up by the anatomist, this uncertainty is not surprising.

Anatomy and melancholy have an affinity; they are both an effect of loss—the loss of meaning, the loss of any clear path to the truth, the loss of power to master an uncertain world. In the anatomies of Lyly, Nashe, Shakespeare, and even Bacon, we find that something is lost that cannot be restored: constancy, coherence, the essences of love and of truth ("a true model of the world"). A melancholy sense that something is lost propels a desire to conduct an anatomy—and anatomy itself creates loss. Anatomy, then, is a cure for melancholy that creates the conditions that produce it. No wonder that Burton endlessly writes his *Anatomy of Melancholy*.

From the outset Burton knows, and does not know, that his method is cause and cure of melancholy. He believes in the power of anatomy as a method for gaining knowledge, yet he also reminds us in the "Preface" that his method of clarification is linked to the undoing of serious, formalizing method with its expectation of making knowledge visible. His task has a "serious intent" and is also a "playing labor." It is a cure for melancholy—"I write of melancholy by being busy to avoid melancholy"—and it sustains melancholy by expanding a mad world of appearances. That mad world is a kind of cure too: the world of illusion is a source of sweetness: the melancholiac feels no fear or sorrow when placed with "phantasms sweet." Much of the *Anatomy of Melancholy* demonstrates the pleasures of a discourse freed from the desire to manifest the truth: "I shall relate things which never have happened and never will happen, merely to show my literary skill . . ." (2.2.58). The *Anatomy*'s digressions, its plethora of contradictory information, the exuberant performance of the preface, the display of melancholy's power of metamorphosis (the power of metaphor itself) which makes Burton's prose almost infinitely rich in stories of transformation are all achievements of the work's subversion of order—and its efforts to discover order. The *Anatomy* remains the equivocal product of both madness and reason. In fact, nothing is conclusive about the *Anatomy* except its lack of conclusion. It ends not because of some internal necessity but because the body of its author fails: only by the accident of Burton's death does the *Anatomy* conclude. But this work does mark another kind of end—the end of anatomy as a popular genre.

Burton's text begins in the unreliable terrain of fragmented words and equivocal meanings—where other anatomies end. It is located at the extreme verge of the form's domain, where reason and madness converge most dramatically. A theological, scientific, and mad work, the *Anatomy of Melancholy* presents the crazy idea never quite spoken by its predecessors: religion, science, and madness may speak the same language. Such a way of unifying the diversity of knowledge is certainly more disconcerting than its compartmentalization. As Foucault writes, "the world of the early seventeenth century [was] strangely hospitable, in all senses, to madness."[20] Later periods were decidedly not. Madness and reason were wrenched apart; institutions were built to contain madmen and positivist doctors attempted to cure madness by silencing it rather than by letting it speak.[21] Anatomy was a mode of writing that had supported the development of a rationalist discourse that could separate truth and falsehood, but because of a paradoxical attachment to the world of appearances, to the uncertainty and excess well demonstrated by Burton's *Anatomy,* it was not the best way to set forth the objective knowledge of the Age of Reason.

Another displaced Anglican divine, Jonathan Swift, adopts the form in *The Tale of a Tub,* but he has as much contempt for his method of exposure as for the contemporary writers he attacks.[22] The voice of the Hack, a persona as unstable as Democritus Junior, has this to say about anatomy:

> And therefore, in order to save the charges of all such expensive anatomy for time to come, I do here think fit to inform the reader, that in such conclusions as these, reason is certainly in the right, and that in most corporeal beings, which have fallen under my cognizance, the outside hath been infinitely preferable to the in; whereof I have been farther convinced from some late experiments. Last week I saw a woman flayed, and you will hardly believe how much it altered her person for the worse. . . . I justly formed this conclusion to myself; that whatever philosopher or projector can find out an art to sodder and patch up the flaws and imperfections of nature, will deserve much better of mankind, and teach us a more useful science, than that so much in present esteem, of widening and exposing them (like him who held anatomy to be the ultimate end of physic).[23]

For Swift, the Hack's modern practice of reason with its emphasis on surfaces and contrived unities is not objective or sane, yet surely the Hack is right about the violent consequences of flaying a body. Not only does an anatomy ruin the human form, the "ultimate end of physic" finally renders bodies as empty as the hollow orders of the projectors. With savage intensity, Swift's *Tale* shows us that the literary anatomy has life in it yet. But for all its power, it is a form without a future: nothing comes of it for the modern scribbler or his opponent. In the eighteenth century, the future of the anatomists' enterprise, their quest to uncover the nature of things, lies in a new form—the novel.

Notes

1 · Of Anatomy

1   For a good introduction to the ideas of Foucault, see his "The Discourse on Language," trans. Rupert Swyer, in *The Archaeology of Knowledge*, trans. A. M. Sheridan Smith (1972; reprint ed., New York: Harper Colophon Books, 1976).

2   In his preface, Reiss offers the simplest explanation of the term "discourse" (he complicates this definition later): "The term 'discourse' refers to the way in which the material embodying sign processes is organized. Discourse can thus be characterized as the visible and describable praxis of what is called 'thinking.' For thinking is nothing but the organization of signs as an ongoing process. Signs themselves may be 'defined' provisionally as the non-discrete 'elements' composing the process toward meaningfulness that itself is both defined by and defining of what signs are" (p.9). Reiss, I will note here, published *The Discourse of Modernism* (Ithaca: Cornell University Press, 1982) after I had finished my work on anatomies, but his brilliant work seems to precede mine. His broad analysis of the emergence and development of Western discourse establishes the domain of language in which the anatomy exists.

3   Readers uncomfortable with such terms as "analytico-referential discourse" will find a cultural crisis narrated in more familiar ways in many other works of Renaissance scholarship such as Hiram Haydn, *The Counter-Renaissance* (New York: Scribners, 1950); Herschel Baker, *The Wars of Truth: Studies in the Decay of Christian Humanism in the Earlier Seventeenth Century* (1952; reprint ed., Gloucester, Mass.: Peter Smith, 1969); and recently, Stephen Greenblatt's *Renaissance Self-Fashioning: From More to Shakespeare* (Chicago and London: University of Chicago Press, 1980).

4   In *The War Against Poetry* (Princeton: Princeton University Press, 1970), Russel Fraser writes, "Medieval man is devoted to the manifold tracings on the surface: the more exclusive impulse that defines his successor is to strike through the mask" (p.44).

5   Charles Singer, *The Evolution of Anatomy: A Short History of Anatomical and Physiological Discovery to Harvey* (New York: A. A. Knopf, 1925), p. 122.

6   Andreas Vesalius, "The Preface of Andreas Vesalius to his Books De humani corporis fabrica addressed to the Divine Charles, Great and Invincible Emperor," *Andreas Vesalius of Brussels 1514–1564,* trans. C. D. O'Malley (Berkeley and Los Angeles: University of California Press, 1964), pp. 320, 319, 323.

7   See Walter Ong's seminal work, *Ramus, Method, and the Decay of Dialogue* (Cambridge: Harvard University Press, 1958); citation from p. 315.

8   In the preface to *The Order of Things: An Archaeology of the Human Sciences,* Alan Sheridan's translation of *Les Mots et Les Choses* (New York: Vintage Books, 1973), Michel Foucault discusses a passage from a Borges story which he says led him to think about knowledge. The passage is supposedly the entry on animals in a Chinese encyclopedia: "animals are divided into: (a) belonging to the Emperor, (b) embalmed, (c) tame, (d) sucking pigs, (e) sirens, (f) fabulous, (g) stray dogs, (h) included in the present classification, (i) frenzied, (j) innumerable . . ." (Borges as cited by Foucault, p. xv). Only the space of the page keeps this menagerie together; there is no thinkable relation among its members. Though the items are ordered by the device of the list, they are not governed by a single order of knowledge.

Renaissance anatomists are also strange list makers. One of them is Thomas Bell, author of *The Anatomie of Popish Tyrannie* (1603). Bell's *Anatomie* contains tables, summaries, and an index that includes the following (page numbers deleted):

Jesuits are great lyers.
Jesuits are cruel tyrants.
Jesuits make a triple vow.
Jesuits are statesmen.
Jesuits ride like Earles.
Jesuits must have their chambers perfumed.
Jesuits are divels.
Jesuits are right Machiavels.
Jesuits are theeves.
Jesuits are proud men.
Jesuits ride in coaches (sig. K).

Though the next entry is not "Jesuits included in the present classification," the list provides its own version of the Chinese encyclopedia's technique by gathering together incongruous attributes under the heading "Jesuit." It does gain unity, however, from the fact that all these attributes are *bad*. Though lists may give the appearance of objectivity, this example undermines the anatomist's claim to a scientific detachment from the material he collects.

9   Galen, *Galen On the Usefulness of the Parts of the Body*, trans. Margaret Tallmadge May (Ithaca: Cornell University Press, 1968), 1:68. In the introduction to *De Usu Partium*, May notes the connection between the soul and Galen's Nature. Nature, she says, "seems something indwelling that controls the organism, or even something apart from it that formed and shaped it in the beginning" (p. 10).

For an account of the relation between microcosm and macrocosm as an analogy that gave a cosmic significance to the body of man, see Leonard Barkan, *Nature's Work of Art: The Human Body as Image of the World* (New Haven and London: Yale University Press, 1975). Barkan, who stresses the "wholeness" and "unity" of Renaissance texts, presents an optimistic view of the artist's ability to create totalities.

10   Andreas Vesalius, "Dedicatory Letter of Vesalius to Phillip II of Spain," *The Epitome of Andreas Vesalius*, trans. L. R. Lind (New York: Macmillan, 1949), p. xxxiv.

11   The identity of the artist responsible for the illustrations of the *Fabrica* has long been disputed. Titian, Jan van Kalkar, Domenico Campagnola, and Vesalius himself have all been credited. See the discussion in J. B. deC. M. Saunders and Charles D. O'Malley, eds., *Illustrations from the Works of Andreas Vesalius of Brussels* (New York: Dover, 1973), pp. 25–29.

12   To know a body, as Foucault has shown, is often to dominate, conquer, master, discipline, and punish it. The science of investigation and surveillance, he says, makes the body an object of knowledge by placing it within a controlled order and separating it into individual elements. See his *Discipline and Punish: The Birth of the Prison*, trans. Alan Sheridan (New York: Pantheon, 1977).

13   I have checked entries in the *Short-Title Catalogue* (Pollard and Redgrave) to determine the earliest of these "spiritual" anatomies. It is possible that I may have missed one that predates Mainardo's *Anatomi*. Other anatomies written from the middle to the turn of the century include: *The Anatomie of the bodie of man*, Thomas Vicary, 1548; *Anatomy of a Hande in the Manner of a Dyall*, Anon., 1554; *Anatomie of the Minde*, Thomas Rogers, 1576; *A Newe Anatomie of Whole Man*, John Woolton, 1576; *Euphues: The Anatomy of Wyt*, John Lyly, 1578; *Valour Anatomized, in a Fancy*, Sir Philip Sidney, 1581; *The Anatomie of Abuses*, Philip Stubbes, 1583; *Anatomy of Lovers' Flatteries*, Robert Greene, 1584; *Arbasto, The Anatomie of Fortune*, Robert Greene, 1584; *The Anatomie of Absurdity*, Thomas Nashe, 1589;

Anatomie of the Metamorphosed Ajax, Sir John Harington, 1596;
A Lively Anatomie of Death, John More, 1596; *The Anatomie of
Pope Joane,* John Mayo, 1597; *The Anatomie of the True Physition and Counterfeit Mountebanke,* Johann Oberndoerffer, 1602;
Anatomie of Sinne, Anon., 1604; *The Anatomie of Popish Tyrannie,* Thomas Bell, 1603; *A New Anatomy,* Robert Underwood,
1605; *Times Anatomie,* Robert Pricket, 1606; *The Anatomie of
Humors,* Simion Grahame, 1609. As Walter Ong notes, the many
other anatomies written at this time are not written in the
vernacular.

Barbara Kiefer Lewalski mentions many of the early, vernacular
anatomies, and adds some later ones, in her discussion of the
anatomy as a form that influenced Donne's "First Anniversarie."
She describes the anatomist as one who analyzes a subject methodi-
cally, often in a denunciatory tone. See her *Donne's Anniversaries
and the Poetry of Praise: The Creation of a Symbolic Mode*
(Princeton: Princeton University Press, 1973), pp. 225–63.

14   Ovid, *Metamorphoses,* 1.1. 190. In *Cony-Catchers and Bawdy
Baskets: An Anthology of Elizabethan Low Life* (Harmondsworth: Penguin, 1972), Gāmini Salgādo translates this quotation
and points out that Robert Greene cites it in both "The Second
Part of Cony-Catching" and "The Defense of Cony-Catching" (see
his note 199).

15   Mainardo, *An Anatomi,* p. 10.

16   John Donne, "The First Anniversarie. An Anatomy of the
World," l. 63, *The Anniversaries,* ed. Frank Manley (Baltimore:
Johns Hopkins University Press, 1963), p. 69.

17   Philip Stubbes, *The Anatomie of Abuses* (London, 1583), p. 10.

18   Ronald Paulson, *Theme and Structure in Swift's Tale of a Tub*
(New Haven: Yale University Press, 1960), p. 7. Paulson believes
Swift parodies anatomies. Denis Donoghue, in *Jonathan Swift: A
Critical Introduction* (London: Cambridge University Press, 1969),
argues that Swift *was* an anatomist. Paulson continues, "But seeking to establish universals, they demonstrate a stronger prob-
ability of nominalism, and their conflict between the validity of
faith and the validity of reason ends with the incidentals col-
lapsing the main argument."

19   See Jacques Derrida, *Of Grammatology,* trans. Gayatri Chakravorty
Spivak (Baltimore and London: Johns Hopkins University Press,
1974), especially the first chapter, "The End of the Book and the
Beginning of Writing."

20   "Epistle Dedicatory to the Novum Organum," *The Philosophical
Works of Francis Bacon,* ed. Robert Ellis and James Spedding
(1857; reprint ed., London: George Routledge and Sons; New
York: E. P. Dutton, 1905), 1:242.

129

21   Paul de Man, "Literary History and Literary Modernity," *Blind-ness and Insight: Essays in the Rhetoric of Contemporary Criticism*
(New York: Oxford University Press, 1971), p. 153.

22   Dan John Tannacito, in his dissertation, "Transformal Structures:
Studies of Anatomy-Romance and Novelistic Romance as Prose
Fictional Genres" (University of Oregon, 1972), says that the
anatomy presents "a parody of the theme of identity" (p. 88). The
obvious example is Democritus Junior in Burton's *Anatomy of*
Melancholy. Nashe presents an earlier example of a writer who
hides behind a screen of extravagant personas.

23   Northrop Frye, *Anatomy of Criticism: Four Essays* (Princeton:
Princeton University Press, 1957), p. 308. Frye was the first to
use the term "anatomy" to define a major category of prose fiction, an "extroverted and intellectual form." The problem with
this classification is that the intellectual displays of the anatomist
are often signs of physical disorders (humors) and the seeming
extroversion of the anatomist is often a means to keep the identity
of the anatomist hidden.

24   Philip Stevick, "Novel and Anatomy: Notes Toward an Amplification of Frye," *Criticism* 10 (Spring 1968): 163. Stevick explains the extroverted nature of the anatomy as a result of the
adoption of oral techniques to the medium of print. Because the
anatomy makes us focus on the materiality and visibility of words,
the explanation seems unsatisfactory. Perhaps it is the printed
condition of the anatomy, not its oral nature, that is responsible
for its "extroversion."

25   See the entries under "anatomy" and "tome" in *An Etymological*
Dictionary of the English Language, ed. Walter W. Skeat (Oxford: Clarendon Press, 1911). "Anatomy" is related to the word
"tome" from the Greek "tomos," which means a piece cut off,
part of a book, a volume (another word suggesting depth, which
has its origin in a roll of paper).

26   Literature, writes Paul de Man, "can be represented as a flight
away from its own specificity and a moment of return to what it
is." See his "Literary History and Literary Modernity," p. 157.

27   *The Notebooks of Leonardo da Vinci,* ed. and trans. Edward Mac-
Curdy (New York: G. Braziller, 1939), 1:188.

28   Robert Burton, *The Anatomy of Melancholy,* ed. Holbrook Jackson (New York: Vintage Books, 1977), p. 15.

2 · *Anatomy as Wit*

1   Charles Baudelaire, "The Painter of Modern Life," *Baudelaire as a*
Literary Critic, trans. Lois Boe Hyslop and Francis E. Hyslop, Jr.
(University Park: Pennsylvania State University Press, 1964),
pp. 299, 297.

2   See R. Warwick Bond's edition of *The Complete Works of John Lyly* (1902; reprint ed., Oxford: Clarendon Press, 1967), 1:160–61, and John Dover Wilson, *John Lyly* (1905; reprint ed., New York: Haskell House, 1970), pp. 80–81.

3   Lyly, *Complete Works*, 1:142.

4   Ibid., p. 71.

5   See G. K. Hunter, *John Lyly: The Humanist as Courtier* (London: Routledge and Kegan Paul, 1962), particularly the first chapter, "Humanism and Courtship."

6   Ibid., p. 276.

7   In the sixteenth century the word "wit" normally referred to the faculty of reason or understanding. The *OED* gives the first recorded use of the word as meaning a "capacity of apt expression" as Lyly's use of the word in *Euphues:* "As the Bee is oftentimes hurt with hir owne Honny, so is witte not seldome plagued with his own conceipt."

8   Jonas Barish, "The Prose Style of John Lyly," *ELH* 23 (1956): 23.

9   All references to the works of John Lyly are to Bond's edition of the *Complete Works*. This quotation is from "Euphues: The Anatomy of Wyt," *Works*, 1:180. I have modernized the spelling of "wyt" to "wit." All citations from Lyly are hereafter referred to by abbreviated name with volume and page number.

10   Though it had a few precursors, Lyly's anatomy had the greatest influence on the anatomies that followed it. *Euphues* was, after all, the most popular book of its time and one of the most self-conscious.

11   Roger Ascham, "The Scholemaster," *English Works*, ed. William Aldis Wright (1904; reprint ed., Cambridge: Cambridge University Press, 1970), p. 214.

12   In his *The Elizabethan Prodigals* (Berkeley and Los Angeles: University of California Press, 1976), Richard Helgerson evinces this distaste: "In the character of Euphues, Lyly created one of the most consistently unsympathetic figures in English literature" (p. 64). Later, he calls Euphues a "monstrous prig." This is itself a somewhat priggish response to the extravagant, contradictory identity of Euphues.

13   See René Girard's seminal work on the structure of "triangular desire," *Deceit, Desire, and the Novel*, trans. Yvonne Freccero (Baltimore and London: Johns Hopkins University Press, 1965).

14   Wilson, *John Lyly*, p. 81.

15   Leon Henry Vincent, *The Bibleotaph, and Other People* (Boston: Houghton Mifflin and Co., 1898), p. 143.

16   Morris Croll, "Introduction," to *Euphues: The Anatomy of Wit* (London: George Routledge and Sons, 1916), p. xvii. Croll wants to separate figures of sound ("schemes") and figures of thought ("tropes") to keep logic and rhetoric separate. Barish ("Prose

Style of John Lyly") shows that Croll's effort to distinguish these
two realms leads to exactly that confusion. By calling a syntactical
structure such as parison "ornamental" and by insisting that a
logical device such as antithesis can be used as a "scheme," Croll,
says Barish, collapses the distinction between rhetoric and logic.
Barish tries to keep them separate by asserting that rhetoric and
logic are indeed equivalent, so form is always meaningful. This
hardly resolves the problem because whether one separates form
and content to protect meaning, or equates form and content to
protect meaning, both actions end up suggesting that "thought
itself is ornamental." I refer readers interested in this problem to
Paul de Man's discussion of the "rhetorization of grammar" in his
article "Semiology and Rhetoric," *Diacritics* 3 (Fall 1973): 27–33.

17 Helgerson, *Elizabethan Prodigals*, p. 61.
18 This question lies at the heart of Helgerson's book.
19 Hunter comments that Lyly's style is "elegant" (*John Lyly*, p. 60)
   and cites an early nineteenth-century critic who remarks on the
   corrupting influence of Euphuism (p. 261). Bond remarks on
   Lyly's love of "adornment" (1:146).
20 Sir Philip Sidney, *The Defense of Poesie*, in *The Prose Works of
   Sir Philip Sidney*, ed. Albert Feuillerat (1922; reprint ed., Cambridge: Cambridge University Press, 1962), 3:42.
21 Ben Jonson, *Every Man Out of His Humor*, in *Ben Jonson*, ed.
   C. H. Herford and Percy Simpson (1927: reprint ed., Oxford:
   Clarendon Press, 1966), 3:490.
22 Hunter, *John Lyly*, p. 257. Rhetoric itself, as Richard Lanham
   has pointed out, was a victim of fashion: "Rhetoric has usually
   been depicted as a woman, especially an overdressed one-harlot
   rhetoric." He goes on to say that "cosmetics, since they are not
   referential, cannot be excessive," nor can style. Like cosmetics,
   style proclaims an attitude. See his excellent discussion of the
   difference between "homo rhetoricus" and "homo serious" in *The
   Motives of Eloquence: Literary Rhetoric in the Renaissance* (New
   Haven: Yale University Press, 1976), pp. 29–30.
23 Edmund Spenser, "Colin Clouts Come Home Againe," *The Works
   of Edmund Spenser: The Minor Poems*, ed. Charles Grosvenor
   Osgood and Henry Gibbons Lotspeich (Baltimore: Johns Hopkins
   University Press, 1949), 3:166.
24 Lyly, *Works*, 1:65.
25 Lawrence Stone, *The Crisis of the Aristocracy 1558–1641*,
   abridged ed. (Oxford and New York: Oxford University Press,
   1967), p. 266.
26 See Hunter, *John Lyly*, p. 285.
27 Friedrich Nietzsche, *The Gay Science*, trans. Walter Kaufmann
   (New York: Vintage Books, 1974), p. 246.

3 · Anatomy as Absurdity

1 G. R. Hibbard, one of the most perceptive of Nashe's critics, remarks that the *Anatomie* "is very much a young man's work and
has little literary merit." He goes on to study the work, however,
because he believes it demonstrates Nashe's early interest in the
medium of prose and the subjects of learning and poetry. See his
Thomas Nashe: A Critical Introduction (London: Routledge and
Kegan Paul, 1962), pp. 10–18.

2 Unfortunately much of my work on anatomies was completed before Jonathan V. Crewe published his excellent discussion of
Nashe's rhetoric: *Unredeemed Rhetoric: Thomas Nashe and the
Scandal of Authorship* (Baltimore and London: Johns Hopkins
University Press, 1982). My citation is from page 25. He calls
attention to Nashe as anatomist in the last sentence of his book:
"If Nashe has fully been recognized as a performer and as a
representative figure of his time, perhaps further recognition is
due to him as a significant anatomist of Elizabethan literary performance" (p. 101). Margaret Ferguson, another sensitive reader
of Nashe, discusses the dangers associated with Nashe's aggressive
verbal skills in an article, "Nashe's *The Unfortunate Traveller:*
The 'Newes of the Maker' Game," *English Literary Renaissance*
2 (Spring 1981): 165–82.

3 Ronald B. McKerrow's introduction to Nashe and his work can
be found in the fifth volume of *The Works of Thomas Nashe*
(1910; reprint ed., Oxford: Basil Blackwell, 1958), pp. 1–34.

4 All citations to Nashe are from *The Works of Thomas Nashe,* ed.
Ronald B. McKerrow. In my text, citations from this edition will
be referred to by an abbreviated title, with volume and page
number.

5 Hibbard, *Thomas Nashe,* p. 180.

6 For the etymology of "absurd" see the entries for the word in
A Concise Etymological Dictionary of the English Language (Ox-
ford: Oxford University Press, 1965) and *The Oxford English
Dictionary.*

7 See Burke's discussion of "Kinds of Reduction" in *A Grammar
of Motives* (Berkeley and Los Angeles: University of California
Press, 1969), pp. 96–101, 506.

8 McKerrow, "Notes," *Works of Thomas Nashe,* 4:2.

9 Edward George Harman, *Gabriel Harvey and Thomas Nashe*
(London: J. M. Ousely, 1923).

10 McKerrow, "Notes," *Works of Thomas Nashe,* 4:1–2.

11 The causes of the quarrel have been examined in detail by Hibbard and McKerrow. Hibbard points out the particular offensive-
ness of Greene's attack on John Harvey. It should be noted that
Nashe had earlier quarreled with Thomas Churchyard—he had

a predilection for verbal bashing (see McKerrow on this topic, ibid., 5:15–16.

12 David Perkins, "Issues and Motivations in the Nashe-Harvey Quarrel," *Philological Quarterly* 39 (April, 1960): 227.

13 Ibid., p. 233.

14 Gabriel Harvey, "Pierces Supererogation," *The Works of Gabriel Harvey,* ed. Alexander B. Grosart (1884–85; reprint ed., New York: AMS Press, 1966), 2:280. Harvey makes this remark in a passage accusing Nashe of disdaining "Thomas Delone, Philip Stubs, Robert Armin" and others because they "hinder his scribling traffique, obscure his resplendishing Fame . . . ," pp. 280–81.

15 Ibid., p. 115.

16 This is Harvey's word for Nashe's style. He gives an example of "pure Nasherie" in "Pierces Supererogation": "Why, thou errant Butter whore, (quoth he, or rather she), thou Cotqueane and scrattop of scolds, wilt thou never leave afflicting a dead carcasse, continually read the Rhetorique Lecture of Ramme ally? A wisp, a wisp, a wisp, ripp, ripp you kitchinstuffe wrangler" (p. 230). The quotation is from *Strange News* (Works, 1:299). Harvey writes later, "God shield quiet men from the handes of such cruell Confuters: whose argumentes are swoordes; whose sentences murthering bullets; whose phrases, crosbarres . . ." (p. 56).

17 Hibbard makes this observation in a discussion of *The Unfortunate Traveller* in *Thomas Nashe,* p. 147. In his "The Lower Style in Nashe's *The Unfortunate Traveller,*" David Kaula attempts to show that this is a style invented only for this late work. I believe Nashe adopted it earlier, but appreciate Kaula's description of Nashe's technique. He says that Nashe's style reveals both a "sheer delight in reproducing the cadences and elegancies of the more artifical styles as an end in itself" and "a searching scepticism toward the attitude implicit in these styles, since they assume a reality more highly ordered and grandiose than is warranted by the elementary facts of experience." See his article in *Studies in English Literature* 6 (Winter 1966): 49.

18 Harvey, "Pierces Supererogation," *Works of Gabriel Harvey,* 2:34.

19 Reprinted by R. B. McKerrow in *Works of Thomas Nashe,* 5:110.

4 · *Anatomy as Comedy*

1 C. L. Barber sets forth his theory of comedy in *Shakespeare's Festive Comedy: A Study of Dramatic Form in Relation to Social Custom* (Princeton: Princeton University Press, 1959). Barber's definition of comic form makes it difficult for him to address the tone of despair and anxiety that characterizes many of the late comedies.

2   From the frontispiece of Thomas Lodge's "Rosalynde. Euphues golden legacie," *The Complete Works of Thomas Lodge* (1883; reprint ed., London: Russell and Russell, 1963), vol. 1.

3   Ibid., pp. 7, 137.

4   All citations from the plays are to *William Shakespeare: The Complete Works,* ed. Alfred Harbage (Baltimore: Penguin, 1970).

5   *King Lear,* I.ii.2–6. In her article "As You Like It" (reprinted in *Shakespeare: The Comedies,* ed. Kenneth Muir [Englewood Cliffs: Prentice-Hall, 1965]), Helen Gardner discusses the elements that relate *As You Like It* to *King Lear.* See especially pp. 65–66.

6   Lyly, *Euphues: The Anatomy of Wit,* in *Works,* 1:195.

7   Roland Barthes, *A Lover's Discourse,* trans. Richard Howard (New York: Hill and Wang, 1978), p. 56.

8   For an analysis of the masque see Angus Fletcher, *The Transcendental Masque: An Essay on Milton's Comus* (Ithaca and London: Cornell University Press, 1971). In his discussion of the ephemerality of the masque and its resort to magic, Fletcher reveals the ambiguous nature of this festive form.

9   Miriam Joseph lists "tautology" as one of the vices of language in her *Shakespeare's Use of the Arts of Language* (New York: Columbia University Press, 1947), p. 302. She also mentions the Tudor rhetoricians' delight in anatomies, a delight shared by Shakespeare (see p. 369).

10   Rosalind chides Orlando because he does not appear to love anyone but himself: "you are rather point-device in your accoustrements, as loving yourself than seeming the lover of any other" (III.ii.360–62).

11   For my understanding of the pastoral I am indebted, as most of us are, to William Empson's *Some Versions of Pastoral* (London: Chatto and Windus, 1935).

12   Touchstone, as has often been noted, here echoes Sir Philip Sidney's remark in *An Apologie for Poetry* that the poet "nothing affirms and therefore never lieth."

13   Perhaps this critique of representation may tell us something about why there are no mothers in *As You Like It* or *King Lear.* Displacements, banishments, exiles can thematize an initial separation from the mother. They also may reveal a desire for such a separation—a desire to avoid natural reproduction and the death and corruption that all living images suffer. In *King Lear* the link between natural reproduction and the horrible fertility of decay underlies the play's most misogynist language.

14   Bridget Gellert Lyons, in *Voice of Melancholy: Studies in Literary Treatments of Melancholy in Renaissance England* (New York: W. W. Norton, 1971), discusses the convention of melancholy in *As You Like It.* Jaques, she says, "gives expression, by his comments

and his very existence, to some of the disharmonies of the forest"
(p. 51).

15 Harold Jenkins suggests a link between Jaques and the studious
middle son of Rowland de Boys, also named Jaques. See his article
"As You Like It," in *Shakespeare Survey* 8, ed. Allardyce Nicoll
(Cambridge: Cambridge University Press, 1955), pp. 40–51.

16 R. Warwick Bond, "Introductory Essay," *Works of John Lyly,"*
p. 167.

5 · *Anatomy as Tragedy*

1 Burckhardt's suggestion that dismemberment is a tragic form of creation was a starting point for my investigation of the play. See his
Shakespearean Meanings (Princeton: Princeton University Press,
1968), p. 15.

2 In *Shakespeare's Imagery and What It Tells Us* (Cambridge: Cambridge University Press, 1965), Caroline Spurgeon points out the
play's obsessive use of verbs and images depicting the human body
in anguished movement (pp. 338–43).

3 John F. Danby, *Shakespeare's Doctrine of Nature* (London: Farber
and Farber, 1949), p. 49. All citations from the play are to *William
Shakespeare: The Complete Works,* ed. Alfred Harbage.

4 Rosalie L. Colie, "The Energies of Endurance: Biblical Echo in King
Lear," in *Some Facets of King Lear,* ed. Rosalie Colie and F. T. Flahiff (Toronto and Buffalo: University of Toronto Press, 1974),
p. 118. Colie also finds comfort in Shakespeare's use of scriptural
language in *King Lear.*

5 Rosalie L. Colie, *Paradoxia Epidemica* (Princeton: Princeton University Press, 1966), p. 7.

6 For an excellent discussion of the role of public exemplum and the
way the movement of the play disrupts such "decorous generaliza-
tion" see James R. Siemon's " 'Turn our impressed lances in our
eyes': Iconoclasm in *King Lear,"* in *Literature and Iconoclasm,* ed.
Brian Caraher and Irving Massey (SUNY Buffalo, 1978), pp. 4–17
and in *Shakespearean Iconoclasm* (Berkeley: University of California Press, forthcoming). Bridget Gellert Lyons in "The Subplot
as Simplification" contrasts the fragmenting experience of the characters in the main plot with the "tendency toward stereotype," in
Colie and Flahiff, *Some Facets of King Lear.*

Both Siemon and Lyons exempt Lear's experience from the limits
of the theater: Siemon by emphasizing Lear's encounter with raw
physical existence located beyond "emblematic schemata" and Lyons
by describing Lear's experience as something greater than literary
forms can express. In my view, Lear's tragedy lies in his inability to
escape from forms that reduce and fragment experience by anatomiz-

ing them—this process of revelation destroys the depths, flattens them out, to make them visible.

7   Angus Fletcher, in *Allegory: The Theory of a Symbolic Mode* (Ithaca and London: Cornell University Press, 1964), explains the way the main protagonists of an allegory generate subcharacters by splitting off aspects of themselves (see pp. 25–29). The splitting off of negative attributes of Lear does not, of course, cleanse him—he remains a character in whom good and evil are mixed.

8   Tolstoy fulminates on the play's incoherence: "But it is not enough that Shakespeare's characters are placed in tragic positions which are impossible, do not flow from the course of events, are inappropriate to time and space—these personages, besides this, act in a way which is out of keeping with their definite character, and is quite arbitrary." See "Shakespeare and the Drama," in *Recollections and Essays,* trans. Aylmer Maude (London and New York: Oxford University Press, 1932), p. 338.

9   A. C. Bradley, *Shakespearean Tragedy* (1904; reprint ed., London: Macmillan, 1964), p. 248.

10 The passage from the *Poetics* that is the root of the ideas of the unity of time reads: "Further, so far as length is concerned tragedy tries as hard as it can to exist during a single daylight period, or to vary but a little . . ." (24). Gerald F. Else, whose translation I use here, notes that this passage does not say "to represent the events of" a single day, so it probably refers to the time it takes to *perform* a tragedy. See Else's commentary on his translation of *Aristotle—Poetics* (Ann Arbor: University of Michigan Press, 1967), p. 89.

11 William R. Elton, *King Lear and the Gods* (San Marino, Calif.: Huntington Library, 1966), p. 330.

12 Ernst H. Kantorowicz, *The King's Two Bodies* (Princeton: Princeton University Press, 1957), p. 40.

13 Roland Barthes, *S/Z,* trans. Richard Miller (New York: Hill and Wang, 1970), pp. 26–27.

14 In this speech Regan unwittingly announces the necessity of a rift between Cornwall and Albany, herself and her sister.

15 In *Discipline and Punish,* trans. Alan Sheridan (New York: Pantheon, 1977), Michel Foucault studies penal methods as expressions of a social order. According to Foucault, before the eighteenth century, punishment was a public spectacle—criminals were tortured, anatomized, to reveal the truth of a crime while simultaneously punishing it. In this ritual, the sovereign affirms his power. By the end of the eighteenth century the spectacle of punishment is hidden, punishment is internalized as social authorities learn to operate on the soul of man.

16 In *The Development of Shakespeare's Imagery* (Cambridge: Harvard Univ. Press, 1951), W. H. Clemen remarks on the infrequent use of imagery in the language of Regan, Goneril, and Edmund.

17 Much has been written on the imagery of sight in *King Lear*. See,

for example, Paul Alpers, "*King Lear* and the Theory of 'The Sight Pattern'," in *In Defense of Reading,* ed. R. Brower and R. Poirer (New York: Dutton, 1963); Stanley Cavell, "The Avoidance of Love: A Reading of *King Lear*," *Must We Mean What We Say* (New York: Charles Scribner's Sons, 1969); Robert B. Heilman, "I Stumbled When I Saw," *This Great Stage: Image and Structure in "King Lear"* (Seattle: University of Washington Press, 1963); and Siemon, " 'Turn our impressed lances'."

18   Laurence Michel, *The Thing Contained: Theory of the Tragic* (Bloomington: Indiana University Press, 1970), p. 164.

19   Mary Claire Randolph, "The Medical Concept in English Renaissance Satiric Theory: Its Possible Relationships and Implications," *Studies in Philology* 38 (April 1941): 125–27.

20   Edmund's deterministic view of nature has the same effect as his father's faith in astrology—it displaces the origin of violence from the human act of interpreting nature to nature itself. But the fact that Edmund's views of nature tell us something about his own character does not mean that they do not also tell us something about the character of nature. In this play the boundaries between inside and outside, between man and nature, are continually violated.

6 · Anatomy as Science

1   Reference to Bacon's writings, with the exception of *The Masculine Birth of Time* and *The Refutation of Philosophies,* are from *The Philosophical Works of Francis Bacon,* vols. 1, 3. Robert Ellis (1857; reprint ed., London: George Routledge and Sons; New York: E. P. Dutton, 1905). Throughout my text, these writings will be referred to by an abbreviated title with volume and page number.

2   Loren C. Eiseley, *The Man Who Saw Through Time* (New York: Charles Scribner's Sons, 1973), p. 70.

3   Thomas Nashe, *The Anatomie of Absurditie,* in *Works,* 1:9.

4   Marshall McLuhan, in "Francis Bacon: Ancient or Modern?" *Renaissance and Reformation* 10 (1974), argues that Bacon approached science "in the spirit of the ancient grammarians and observers of the page of nature . . ." (p. 94).

5   As Puritan beliefs in man's wickedness encouraged movements of reformation, so Bacon's view of man's limitations compelled him to devise a method for overcoming those limitations and establishing a new order on earth.

6   C. S. Lewis says of Bacon that he is best "not as discoverer of truths but as exposer of fallacies." See his *English Literature in the Sixteenth Century Excluding Drama* (Oxford: Clarendon Press, 1954), p. 537. Bacon does not spare "anatomy" when exposing the limits of methods of knowledge: in the *Advancement* he complains that

anatomists have not discovered all the secrets of the body because few live anatomies are performed. He is also aware that anatomists tend to be overly fascinated with parts.

7   Francis Bacon, *The Masculine Birth of Time,* in *The Philosophy of Francis Bacon,* trans. Benjamin Farrington (Liverpool: Liverpool University Press, 1964), p. 70.

8   Reiss, *Discourse of Modernism,* p. 189.

9   Lisa Jardine makes a similar observation in *Francis Bacon: Discovery and the Art of Discourse* (London: Cambridge University Press, 1974), p. 96.

10   Brian Vickers remarks that "Bacon's increasing use of natural, organic imagery for knowledge . . . modifies the implications of an 'anatomy,' for instead of a cutting-up of nature we are presented with the idea of division as being a temporary highlighting of a branch within the fundamental unity of the sciences." See his *Francis Bacon and Renaissance Prose* (Cambridge: Cambridge University Press, 1968), p. 58.

11   Foucault, *The Order of Things,* pp. 54–55.

12   See Stanley E. Fish, *Self-Consuming Artifacts: The Experience of Seventeenth-Century Literature* (Berkeley and Los Angeles: University of California Press, 1972), pp. 78–144.

13   Paoli Rossi, *Francis Bacon: From Magic to Science,* trans. Sacha Rabinovitch (Chicago: University of Chicago Press, 1968), p. 182.

14   Jardine, *Francis Bacon,* p. 176.

15   Bacon, *The Masculine Birth of Time,* p. 68.

16   Reiss, *Discourse of Modernism,* p. 194.

17   Timothy Reiss, "Introduction: The Word/World Equation," *Yale French Studies* 49 (1973): 6.

18   Hugo von Hofmannsthal, "The Letter of Lord Chandos," in *Selected Prose,* trans. Mary Hottinger, Tania Stern, and James Stern (New York: Pantheon, 1952), pp. 132, 134.

19   Francis Bacon, *The Refutation of Philosophies,* in *Philosophy of Francis Bacon,* p. 132.

7 · *Anatomy as Reason and Madness*

1   Ruth A. Fox, *The Tangled Chain: The Structure of Disorder in the Anatomy of Melancholy* (Berkeley and Los Angeles: University of California Press, 1976), pp. 39–40. Fox insists that Burton's work is a cure for melancholy because it is "art" that bestows on its parts an "organic" unity (pp. 9, 272). But everywhere she reveals Burton's text to be full of contradictions that can only be given a coherent meaning by insisting that the form of the book binds its numerous parts into a single, idealized object. While her interpretation allows us to feel that Burton is almost a god because his text can contain everything within a sublime order, this explanation will not satisfy

the reader who marvels not at the work's totality but at its openness, its mad refusal to make any truth the ultimate one. For a brilliant discussion of the critical practice of shaping texts into objects of the reader's awe, see William Beatty Warner's discussion of the "humanist sublime" in his *Reading Clarissa: The Struggles of Interpretation* (New Haven and London: Yale University Press, 1979), pp. 241–56.

2   The range of responses to Burton's work extends from William Osler's view of the text as a "great medical treatise, orderly in arrangement" ("Burton's *Anatomy of Melancholy*," *Yale Review* 3 [1914]: 252) to Stanley Fish's insistence that unreliability is normal in the *Anatomy:* "nonmethod" is "methodized" ("Democritus Jr. to the Reader," in *Self-Consuming Artifacts,* p. 332).

3   Lawrence Babb, *Sanity in Bedlam: A Study of Robert Burton's "Anatomy of Melancholy"* (East Lansing: Michigan State University Press, 1959); Ruth Fox, *The Tangled Chain;* James Roy King, "The Genesis of Burton's Anatomy of Melancholy," in *Studies in Six 17th Century Writers* (Athens: Ohio University Press, 1966), p. 59.

4   Osler, "Burton's *Anatomy of Melancholy*," p. 252.

5   All my citations from the *Anatomy* are to Robert Burton, *Anatomy of Melancholy,* ed. with an introduction by Holbrook Jackson. Each citation includes partition, section, and page number. Citations from the "Preface" are marked P with page number included. Brackets within quotations are those provided by Jackson except for my explanation of the pronoun, in the citation from 1.2.177–78.

6   Jean Starobinski, "La Mélancolie de l'Anatomiste," *Tel Quel* 10 (1962): 22. A translation of the passage is "This melancholy clergyman has perfectly demonstrated the desperate and despairing aspect of all that has been called science up to the present: the accumulation and juxtaposition of this wisdom manifests a secret madness."

7   I use Fox's terminology here. See *The Tangled Chain,* p. 8.

8   David Renaker, "Robert Burton and Ramist Method," *Renaissance Quarterly* 24 (1971): 212.

9   Ibid., p. 219.

10 David Renaker, "Robert Burton's Tricks of Memory," *PMLA* 87 (1972): 393.

11 F. P. Wilson, "Robert Burton," in *Seventeenth Century Prose: Five Lectures* (Berkeley and Los Angeles: University of California Press, 1960), p. 34. Wilson quotes a passage in which Burton's praise of fishing really belongs to "a 'Treatise of Fishing with an Angle' printed by Wynkyn de Worde as early as 1496."

12 Fish, *Self-Consuming Artifacts,* p. 329.

13 See Joan Webber, *The Eloquent "I": Style and Self in Seventeenth-Century Prose* (Madison: University of Wisconsin Press, 1968). See also Rosalie Colie's discussion of the *Anatomy of Melancholy* in *Paradoxia Epidemica* (Princeton: Princeton University Press, 1966)

and Bridget Gellert Lyons, *Voices of Melancholy: Studies in Literary Treatments of Melancholy in Renaissance England* (New York: W. W. Norton, 1971).

14   In "Training his Melancholy Spaniel: Persona and Structure in Robert Burton's 'Democritus Jr. to the Reader'," *Philological Quarterly* 55 (1976), Reinhard H. Friederich discusses how Burton developed his persona to demonstrate and exemplify a melancholy world.

15   Robert Burton, *Anatomy of Melancholy*, "The Conclusion of the Author to the Reader" (Oxford, 1621), Ddd I.

16   Fish, *Self-Consuming Artifacts*, p. 306.

17   The connection between madness and the sea, symbolized in the *Ship of Fools*, is an old one. Burton uses the metaphors of the sea frequently in his descriptions of the space of melancholy. Here is a good example: "Give me but a little leave, and I will set before your eyes in brief a stupend, vast, infinite ocean of incredible madness and folly: a sea full of shelves and rocks, sands, gulfs, euripes and contrary tides, full of fearful monsters, uncouth shapes, roaring waves, tempests, and siren calms, halcyonian seas, unspeakable misery, such comedies and tragedies, such absurd and ridiculous, feral and lamentable fits . . ." (3.4.313).

18   Michel Foucault, *Madness and Civilization: A History of Insanity in the Age of Reason*, trans. Richard Howard (New York: Pantheon, 1973), p. 213.

19   William Mueller, *The Anatomy of Robert Burton's England* (Berkeley and Los Angeles: University of California Press, 1952), p. 85. See also Robert M. Browne, "Robert Burton and the New Cosmology," *Modern Language Quarterly* 13 (1952) and Richard Barlow, "Infinite Worlds: Robert Burton's Cosmic Voyage," *Journal of the History of Ideas* 34 (1973). See also Marjorie Hope Nicolson, *The Breaking of the Circle: Studies in the Effect of the "New Science" upon Seventeenth Century Poetry*, rev. ed. (New York: Columbia University Press, 1960).

20   Foucault, *Madness and Civilization*, p. 37.

21   The story of the classical experience and treatment of madness is narrated by Foucault, ibid.

22   As I pointed out in an earlier note (chap. 1, n.18), Ronald Paulson believes that Swift parodied anatomies and Denis Donoghue thinks that Swift wrote in earnest. Edward Said in *Beginnings: Intention and Method* (New York: Basic Books, 1975) describes Swift's writing in terms that could easily be attached to Burton: the narrator/author of Swift's *Tale of a Tub* is "perhaps the most thoroughly imagined bibliomyth ever produced" and later "Swift [is] extraordinarily addicted to quotation" (pp. 21–22). Frank Kinahan, in "The Melancholy of Anatomy: Voice and Theme in *A Tale of a Tub*," *Journal of English and German Philology* 69 (1970), suggests that the moderns are anatomists: "When the Hack praises the divi-

sion of knowledge into systems, abstracts, and indexes, what he is really doing is describing other sorts of skeletons. The moderns seem to themselves to be moving through ordering to knowledge but what they are in fact doing is rendering knowledge impossible by emptying out the objects of knowledge" (p. 289). Reiss points out that Swift is writing after the discourse of patterning has "yielded completely" to the dominance of analytico-referential discourse—he doesn't, then, have all the stylistic choices available to him that Burton does. See Reiss, *Discourse of Modernism,* pp. 328–57.

23 Jonathan Swift, *Gulliver's Travels and Other Writings,* ed. Louis A. Landa (London and Oxford: Oxford University Press, 1976), p. 333. Swift doesn't call his work an anatomy perhaps because he hopes his satiric purposes will distance him from all forms. His work is, however, bounded by the forms he must work within.

Works Cited

Ackerman, James. "On Scientia." In *Science and Culture: A Study of Cohesive and Disjunctive Forces,* edited by Gerald Holton. Boston: Beacon Press, 1965.

Alpers, Paul J. "*King Lear* and the Theory of 'The Sight Pattern'." In *In Defense of Reading,* edited by Reuben A. Brower and Richard Poirer. New York: Dutton, 1962.

Anatomy of a Hande in the Manner of a Dyall. London, 1554.

Anatomy of Sinne, 1604.

Aristotle. *Aristotle—Poetics.* Translated by Gerald F. Else. Ann Arbor: University of Michigan Press, 1967.

Ascham, Roger. "The Scholemaster." *English Works.* Edited by William Aldis Wright. 1904. Reprint. Cambridge: Cambridge University Press, 1970.

Babb, Lawrence. *Sanity in Bedlam: A Study of Robert Burton's "Anatomy of Melancholy."* East Lansing: Michigan State University Press, 1959.

Bacon, Francis. *The Complete Works of Francis Bacon.* Edited by James Spedding, Robert Ellis, and Douglas D. Heath. Vol. 3. London: Longman and Co., 1889.

————. *The Masculine Birth of Time* and *The Refutation of Philosophies. The Philosophy of Francis Bacon.* Translated by Benjamin Farrington. Liverpool: Liverpool University Press, 1964.

————. *The Philosophical Works of Francis Bacon.* Edited by Robert Ellis and James Spedding. 1857. Reprint. London: George Routledge and Sons; New York: E. P. Dutton, 1905.

Baker, Herschel. *The Wars of Truth: Studies in the Decay of Christian Humanism in the Earlier Seventeenth Century.* 1952. Reprint. Gloucester, Mass.: Peter Smith, 1969.

Barber, C. L. *Shakespeare's Festive Comedy: A Study of Dramatic Form in Relation to Social Custom.* Princeton: Princeton University Press, 1959.

Barish, Jonas. "The Prose Style of John Lyly." *ELH* 23 (1956): 14–35.

Barkan, Leonard. *Nature's Work of Art: The Human Body as Image of the World.* New Haven and London: Yale University Press, 1975.

Barlow, Richard G. "Infinite Worlds: Robert Burton's Cosmic Voyage." *Journal of the History of Ideas* 34 (1973): 291–302.

Barthes, Roland. *A Lover's Discourse.* Translated by Richard Howard. New York: Hill and Wang, 1978.

———. "Science versus Literature." In *Introduction to Structuralism,* edited by Michael Lane. New York: Basic Books, 1970.

———. *S/Z.* Translated by Richard Miller. New York: Hill and Wang, 1970.

Baudelaire, Charles. "The Painter of Modern Life." In *Baudelaire as a Literary Critic.* Translated by Lois Boe Hyslop and Francis E. Hyslop, Jr. University Park: Pennsylvania State University Press, 1964.

Bell, Thomas. *The Anatomie of Popish Tyrannie.* London, 1603.

Bradley, A. C. *Shakespearean Tragedy.* 1904. Reprint. London: Macmillan, 1964.

Browne, Robert M. "Robert Burton and the New Cosmology." *Modern Language Quarterly* 13 (1952): 131–48.

Burckhardt, Sigurd. *Shakespearean Meanings.* Princeton: Princeton University Press, 1968.

Burke, Kenneth. *A Grammar of Motives.* Berkeley and Los Angeles: University of California Press, 1969.

Burton, Robert. *The Anatomy of Melancholy: What it is with all the kinds, causes, symptomes, prognostickes and severall cures of it.* Edited by Holbrook Jackson. New York: Vintage Books, 1977.

Cavell, Stanley. "The Avoidance of Love: A Reading of *King Lear.*" In *Must We Mean What We Say?* New York: Charles Scribner's Sons, 1969.

Clemen, W. H. *The Development of Shakespeare's Imagery.* Cambridge: Harvard University Press, 1951.

Colie, Rosalie L. "The Energies of Endurance." In *Some Facets of King Lear,* edited by Rosalie L. Colie and F. T. Flahiff. Toronto and Buffalo: University of Toronto Press, 1974.

———. *Paradoxia Epidemica.* Princeton: Princeton University Press, 1966.

Crewe, Jonathan V. *Unredeemed Rhetoric: Thomas Nashe and the Scandal of Authorship.* Baltimore and London: Johns Hopkins University Press, 1982.

Croll, Morris. Introduction, to *Euphues: The Anatomy of Wit.* Edited by Morris Croll and Harry Clemons. London: George Routledge and Sons, 1916.

Danby, John F. *Shakespeare's Doctrine of Nature.* London: Farber and Farber, 1949.

de Man, Paul. "Literary History and Literary Modernity." In *Blindness and Insight: Essays in the Rhetoric of Contemporary Criticism.* New York: Oxford University Press, 1971.

————. "Semiology and Rhetoric." *Diacritics* 3 (Fall 1973): 27–33.

Derrida, Jacques. *Of Grammatology.* Translated by Gayatri Chakravorty Spivak. Baltimore and London: Johns Hopkins University Press, 1974.

Donne, John. "The First Anniversarie. An Anatomy of the World." *The Anniversaries.* Edited by Frank Manley. Baltimore: Johns Hopkins University Press, 1963.

Donoghue, Denis. *Jonathan Swift: A Critical Introduction.* London: Cambridge University Press, 1969.

Eiseley, Loren C. *The Man Who Saw Through Time.* New York: Charles Scribner's Sons, 1973.

Elton, William R. *King Lear and the Gods.* San Marino, Calif.: Huntington Library, 1966.

Empson, William. *Some Versions of Pastoral.* London: Chatto and Windus, 1935.

Ferguson, Margaret. "Nashe's *The Unfortunate Traveller:* The 'Newes of the Maker' Game." *English Literary Renaissance* 2 (Spring 1981): 165–82.

Fish, Stanley E. *Self-Consuming Artifacts: The Experience of Seventeenth-Century Literature.* Berkeley and Los Angeles: University of California Press, 1972.

Fletcher, Angus. *Allegory: The Theory of a Symbolic Mode.* Ithaca and London: Cornell University Press, 1964.

————. *The Transcendental Masque: An Essay on Milton's Comus.* Ithaca and London: Cornell University Press, 1971.

Foucault, Michel. *Discipline and Punish: The Birth of the Prison.* Translated by Alan Sheridan. New York: Pantheon, 1977.

————. "The Discourse on Language," trans. Rupert Swyer. In *The Archaeology of Knowledge.* Translated by A. M. Sheridan Smith. 1972. Reprint. New York: Harper Colophon Books, 1976.

————. *Madness and Civilization: A History of Insanity in the Age of Reason.* Translated by Richard Howard. New York: Pantheon, 1973.

————. *The Order of Things: An Archaeology of the Human Sciences* (a translation of *Les Mots et les Choses*). Translated by Alan Sheridan. New York: Vintage Books, 1973.

Fox, Ruth A. *The Tangled Chain: The Structure of Disorder in the Anatomy of Melancholy.* Berkeley and Los Angeles: University of California Press, 1976.

Fraser, Russel. *The War Against Poetry.* Princeton: Princeton University Press, 1970.

Friederich, Reinhard H. "Training his Melancholy Spaniel: Persona and Structure in Robert Burton's 'Democritus Junior to the Reader.'" *Philological Quarterly* 55 (1976): 195–210.

Frye, Northrop. *Anatomy of Criticism: Four Essays.* Princeton: Princeton University Press, 1957.

Galen. *Galen On the Usefulness of the Parts of the Body.* Translated by

Margaret Tallmadge May. Vol. 1. Ithaca: Cornell University Press, 1968.

Gardner, Helen. "As You Like It." In *Shakespeare: The Comedies*. Edited by Kenneth Muir. Englewood Cliffs: Prentice-Hall, 1965.

Gilbert, Neal W. *Renaissance Concepts of Method*. New York: Columbia University Press, 1960.

Girard, René. *Deceit, Desire, and the Novel*. Translated by Yvonne Freccero. Baltimore and London: Johns Hopkins University Press, 1965.

Grahame, Simion. *The Anatomie of Humors*. Edinburgh, 1609.

Greenblatt, Stephen. *Renaissance Self-Fashioning: From More to Shakespeare*. Chicago and London: University of Chicago Press, 1980.

Greene, Robert. *Anatomy of Lovers' Flatteries*. London, 1584.

———. *Arbasto: The Anatomie of Fortune*. London, 1584.

Harman, Edward George. *Gabriel Harvey and Thomas Nashe*. London: J. M. Ousley, 1923.

Harington, John. *Anatomie of the Metamorphosed Ajax*. London, 1596.

Harvey, Gabriel. "Pierces Supererogation." *The Works of Gabriel Harvey*. Edited by Alexander B. Grosart. Vol. 2. 1884–85. Reprint. New York: AMS Press, 1966.

Haydn, Hiram. *The Counter-Renaissance*. New York: Scribners, 1950.

Heilman, Robert B. *This Great Stage: Image and Structure in "King Lear."* Seattle: University of Washington Press, 1963.

Helgerson, Richard. *The Elizabethan Prodigals*. Berkeley and Los Angeles: University of California Press, 1976.

Hibbard, G. R. *Thomas Nashe: A Critical Introduction*. London: Routledge and Kegan Paul, 1962.

Hunter, G. K. *John Lyly: The Humanist as Courtier*. London: Routledge and Kegan Paul, 1962.

Jardine, Lisa. *Francis Bacon: Discovery and the Art of Discourse*. London: Cambridge University Press, 1974.

Jenkins, Harold. "As You Like It." In *Shakespeare Survey 8,* edited by Allardyce Nicoll. Cambridge: Cambridge University Press, 1955.

Jonson, Ben. *Every Man Out of His Humor. Ben Jonson*. Edited by C. H. Herford and Percy Simpson. Vol. 3. 1927. Reprint. Oxford: Clarendon Press, 1966.

Joseph, Miriam. *Shakespeare's Use of the Arts of Language*. New York: Columbia University Press, 1947.

Kantorowicz, Ernst H. *The King's Two Bodies*. Princeton: Princeton University Press, 1957.

Kaula, David. "The Lower Style in Nashe's *The Unfortunate Traveller."* *Studies in English Literature* 6 (Winter 1966): 43–57.

Kinahan, Frank. "The Melancholy of Anatomy: Voice and Theme in *A Tale of a Tub." Journal of English and German Philology* 69 (1970): 278–91.

King, James Roy. "The Genesis of Burton's Anatomy of Melancholy." In *Studies in Six 17th Century Writers*. Athens: Ohio University Press, 1966.

Lanham, Richard. *The Motives of Eloquence: Literary Rhetoric in the Renaissance.* New Haven: Yale University Press, 1976.

Leonardo da Vinci. *The Notebooks of Leonardo da Vinci.* Edited and translated by Edward MacCurdy. New York: G. Braziller, 1939.

Lewalski, Barbara Kiefer. *Donne's Anniversaries and the Poetry of Praise: The Creation of a Symbolic Mode.* Princeton: Princeton University Press, 1973.

Lewis, C. S. *English Literature in the Sixteenth Century Excluding Drama.* Oxford: Clarendon Press, 1954.

Lodge, Thomas. "Rosalynde. Euphues golden legacie." *The Complete Works of Thomas Lodge.* Vol. 1. 1883. Reprint. London: Russell and Russell, 1963.

Lyly, John. *The Complete Works of John Lyly.* Edited by R. Warwick Bond. Vol. 1. 1902. Reprint. Oxford: Clarendon Press, 1967.

Lyons, Bridget Gellert. "The Subplot as Simplification." In *Some Facets of King Lear,* edited by Rosalie Colie and F. T. Flahiff. Toronto and Buffalo: University of Toronto Press, 1974.

——. *Voices of Melancholy: Studies in Literary Treatments of Melancholy in Renaissance England.* New York: W. W. Norton, 1971.

Mainardo, Augustino. *An Anatomi: that is to say a parting in pieces of the Mass.* Strasburg[?], 1556.

McLuhan, Marshall. "Francis Bacon: Ancient or Modern?" *Renaissance and Reformation* 10 (1974): 93–98.

Mayo, John. *The Anatomie of Pope Joane.* London: 1597.

Michel, Laurence. *The Thing Contained: Theory of the Tragic.* Bloomington: Indiana University Press, 1970.

More, John. *A Livelie Anatomie of Death.* London, 1596.

Mueller, William. *The Anatomy of Robert Burton's England.* Berkeley and Los Angeles: University of California Press, 1952.

Nashe, Thomas. *The Works of Thomas Nashe.* Edited by Ronald B. McKerrow. Vols. 1, 3, 5. 1904–1910. Reprint. Oxford: Basil Blackwell, 1958.

Nietzsche, Friedrich. *The Gay Science.* Translated by Walter Kaufman. New York: Vintage Books, 1974.

Nicolson, Marjorie Hope. *The Breaking of the Circle: Studies in the Effect of the "New Science" upon Seventeenth Century Poetry.* Rev. ed. New York: Columbia University Press, 1960.

Oberndoerffer, Johann. *The Anatomie of the True Physition and Counterfeit Mountebanke.* London, 1602.

Ong, Walter, J. *Ramus, Method, and the Decay of Dialogue.* Cambridge: Harvard University Press, 1958.

Osler, William. "Burton's *Anatomy of Melancholy.*" *Yale Review* 3 (1914): 251–71.

Paulson, Ronald. *Theme and Structure in Swift's Tale of a Tub.* New Haven: Yale University Press, 1960.

Perkins, David. "Issues and Motivations in the Nashe–Harvey Quarrel." *Philological Quarterly* 39 (April 1960): 224–33.

Pricket, Robert. *Times Anatomie*. London, 1606.

Randolph, Mary Claire. "The Medical Concept in English Renaissance Satiric Theory: Its Possible Relationships and Implications." *Studies in Philology* 38 (April 1941): 125–57.

Reiss, Timothy J. *The Discourse of Modernism*. Ithaca: Cornell University Press, 1982.

———. "Introduction: The Word/World Equation." *Yale French Studies* 49 (1973): 3–12.

Renaker, David. "Robert Burton and Ramist Method." *Renaissance Quarterly* 24 (1971): 210–20.

———. "Robert Burton's Tricks of Memory." *PMLA* 87 (1972): 391–96.

Rogers, Thomas. *Anatomie of the Minde*. London, 1576.

Rossi, Paoli. *Francis Bacon: From Magic to Science*. Translated by Sacha Rabinovitch. Chicago: University of Chicago Press, 1968.

Said, Edward. *Beginnings: Intention and Method*. New York: Basic Books, 1975.

Salgādo, Gāmini, ed. *Cony-Catchers and Bawdy Baskets: An Anthology of Elizabethan Low Life*. Harmondsworth: Penguin, 1972.

Saunders, J. B. deC. M., and O'Malley, C. D., eds. *Illustrations from the Works of Andreas Vesalius of Brussels*. New York: Dover, 1973.

Shakespeare, William. *The Complete Pelican Shakespeare*. Edited by Alfred Harbage. New York: Viking Press, 1969.

Sidney, Sir Philip. "The Defense of Poesie." *The Prose Works of Sir Philip Sidney*. Edited by Albert Feuillerat. Cambridge: Cambridge University Press, 1962.

———. *Valour Anatomized, in a Fancy*. London, 1581.

Siemon, James R. " 'Turn our impressed lances in our eyes': Iconoclasm in *King Lear*." In *Literature and Iconoclasm,* edited by Brian Caraher and Irving Massey. *SUNY* Buffalo, 1978.

Singer, Charles. *The Evolution of Anatomy: A Short History of Anatomical and Physiological Discovery to Harvey*. New York: A. A. Knopf, 1925.

Skeat, Walter W., ed. *An Etymological Dictionary of the English Language*. Oxford: Clarendon Press, 1911.

Spenser, Edmund. "Colin Clouts Come Home Againe." *The Works of Edmund Spenser*. Edited by Charles Grosvenor Osgood and Henry Gibbons Lotspeich. Vol. 3. Baltimore: Johns Hopkins University Press, 1949.

Spurgeon, Caroline. *Shakespeare's Imagery and What It Tells Us*. Cambridge: Cambridge University Press, 1965.

Starobinski, Jean. "La Mélancolie de l'Anatomiste." *Tel Quel* 10 (1962): 21–29.

Stevick, Philip. "Novel and Anatomy: Notes toward an Amplification of Frye." *Criticism* 10 (Spring 1968): 153–65.

Stone, Lawrence. *The Crisis of the Aristocracy 1558–1641*. Abridged ed. London and Oxford: Oxford University Press, 1967.

Stubbes, Philip. *The Anatomie of Abuses.* London, 1583.

Swift, Jonathan. *Gulliver's Travels and Other Writings.* Edited by Louis A. Landa. London and Oxford: Oxford University Press, 1976.

Tannacito, Dan John. "Transformal Structures: Studies of Anatomy-Romance and Novelistic Romance as Prose Fictional Genres." Ph.D. diss., University of Oregon, 1972.

Tolstoy, Leo. "Shakespeare and the Drama." *Recollections and Essays.* Translated by Aylmer Maude. London and New York: Oxford University Press, 1932.

Underwood, Robert. *A New Anatomy.* London, 1605.

Vesalius, Andreas. "Dedicatory Letter of Vesalius to Phillip II of Spain." *The Epitome of Andreas Vesalius.* Translated by L. R. Lind. New York: Macmillan, 1949.

————. "The Preface of Andreas Vesalius to his Books De humani corporis fabrica addressed to the Divine Charles, Great and Invincible Emperor." *Andreas Vesalius of Brussels 1514–1564.* Translated by C. D. O'Malley. Berkeley and Los Angeles: University of California Press, 1964.

Vicary, Thomas. *The Anatomie of the bodie of man.* London, 1548.

Vickers, Brian. *Francis Bacon and Renaissance Prose.* Cambridge: Cambridge University Press, 1968.

Vincent, Leon Henry. *The Bibleotaph, and Other People.* Boston: Houghton Mifflin and Co., 1898.

Von Hofmannsthal, Hugo. "Letter of Lord Chandos." *Selected Prose.* Translated by Mary Hottinger, Tania Stern, and James Stern. New York: Pantheon, 1952.

Warner, William Beatty. *Reading Clarissa: The Struggles of Interpretation.* New Haven and London: Yale University Press, 1979.

Webber, Joan. *The Eloquent "I": Style and Self in Seventeenth-Century Prose.* Madison: University of Wisconsin Press, 1968.

Wilson, F. P. *Seventeenth Century Prose.* Berkeley and Los Angeles: University of California Press, 1960.

Wilson, John Dover. *John Lyly.* 1905. Reprint. New York: Haskell House, 1970.

Woolton, John. *A Newe Anatomie of Whole Man.* London, 1576.

Index